COST-EFFECTIVE NURSING PRACTICE: Guidelines for Nurse Managers

Philadelphia   **J. B. LIPPINCOTT COMPANY**

London   Mexico City   New York   St. Louis   São Paulo   Sydney

COST-EFFECTIVE NURSING PRACTICE: Guidelines for Nurse Managers

Doris R. Blaney, R.N., Ed.D., F.A.A.N.

Assistant Dean and Professor of Nursing
Indiana University School of Nursing (Northwest Campus),
and Chairman, Division of Nursing
Indiana University Northwest,
Gary, Indiana

Charles J. Hobson, Ph.D.

Associate Professor of Management and Personnel
Division of Business and Economics
Indiana University Northwest
Gary, Indiana

CONTRIBUTOR: Joseph Scodro, M.B.A., C.P.A.

Assistant Professor of Accounting
Division of Business and Economics
Indiana University Northwest
Gary, Indiana

Sponsoring Editor: Nancy Mullins
Manuscript Editor: Marjory I. Fraser
Indexer: Nancy Weaver
Design Coordinator: Anita R. Curry
Production Manager: Kathleen P. Dunn
Production Coordinator: Fred D. Wood IV
Compositor: Digitype, Inc.
Printer/Binder: R. R. Donnelley & Sons, Company

6   5   4   3   2   1

Library of Congress Cataloging-in-Publication Data

Blaney, Doris R.
  Cost-effective nursing practice.

  Includes index.
    1. Nursing — Cost effectiveness.   2. Nursing
services — Administration.   I. Hobson, Charles J.
II. Title. [DNLM: 1. Administrative Personnel.
2. Cost Benefit Analysis — nurses' instruction.
3. Economics, Nursing.   WY 77 B642c]
RT86.7.B57   1988   362.1'73'0681   87-31068
ISBN 0-397-54649-1

The price a family pays for an author's book is high. Our family members put up with our obsessions and unpredictable work habits. We express our gratitude and indebtedness by dedicating this book to them.

To Bob — For all his love, support, and encouragement; to Jim, Sue, and Tom for enriching my life in so many special ways; and to the memory of my parents, Elnora and Frank Papke, who believed in and supported me in all my endeavors.

To Gabi — For all of her love, hard work, parenting, and dedication; to Natalie and Josh for all the joy and happiness they have brought me; to Mom and Dad for all of the advice, opportunities, and support they have provided over the years.

Preface

The purpose of *Cost-Effective Nursing Practice: Guidelines for Nurse Managers* is to provide nurses with the skills necessary to improve the cost-effectiveness of the patient care process while improving quality. These skills include an understanding of the important motivational/attitudinal factors, along with a thorough grasp of specific management techniques designed to control costs and improve productivity.

Nurses who will find this book useful include:

1. Nurses in supervisory/management positions, from head nurses up
2. Nurses who plan to become managers
3. Staff nurses concerned with cost control
4. Students in baccalaureate programs (*i.e.*, supplemental text in Management/Leadership courses)
5. Students in graduate programs (*i.e.*, Nursing Administration major)
6. Nursing faculty

The book briefly examines the current situation in health care and identifies nursing's pivotal role in improving cost-effectiveness. Important attitudinal factors are addressed in Section One, and practical, research proven management techniques are introduced in Section Two to help nurses improve the cost-effectiveness and quality of patient care. The book concludes with a discussion of future trends in nursing.

The major strengths of the book include the following:

1. The straightforward application of research tested and proven business techniques and strategies to reduce costs and improve quality
   - Goal setting in patient teaching

- ▪ The critical path method in scheduling
- ▪ Efficient use of supplies

2. A unifying conceptual model of the nurse's pivotal and powerful position in the drive to reduce costs

3. A simple formula that tells us that a person's performance is a function of two major factors: ability and motivation

4. A chapter on power in nursing and how to enhance it

5. A consideration of proven approaches to enhance nursing attitudes and motivation

6. A practical style, with emphasis on implementing and using new approaches

7. An emphasis on working smarter, not harder, to control costs and improve quality

8. Convenient chapter summaries of major points

9. Actual nursing examples to illustrate key concepts

Readers will (1) better understand the current crisis in health care and the personal and professional implications; (2) realize the critical role nursing occupies in responding to the challenges of cost control; (3) appreciate the importance of motivational/attitudinal factors in determining nursing success and learn approaches to improve in these areas; and (4) learn specific, research-tested, and practical procedures to cut costs, while improving the quality of care.

Our book is important because it represents the application of practical business management techniques in nursing to control costs. It puts nurses in the pivotal position to control costs and provides the profession with a major challenge and opportunity to excel.

Doris R. Blaney, R.N., Ed.D., F.A.A.N.
Charles J. Hobson, Ph.D.

Acknowledgments

Since early 1984, when we began our research on cost-effective nursing practices at The Methodist Hospitals of Gary and Merrillville, Indiana, we have been both impressed and pleased with the cooperation of the staff at the agency.

We are especially grateful to John Betjemann, Corporate President, and Sherry Burger, Corporate Vice-President of Nursing Services, for encouraging us and giving us considerable support to conduct our research. They provided an environment that promoted an excellent opportunity for us to proceed efficiently and effectively.

We also want to thank the following individuals for all their assistance with our research:

*Dolores Williams, R.N.

Marlene Hedges, R.N.

Dave Parry

*Liz Elich, R.N.

Joan Sohaney

*Judy Berg, R.N.

*Dolores Pictor, R.N.

*Debbie Drescher, R.N.

Directors and Assistant Directors

Experimental Units

*Jennifer Whitfield, R.N.

Karen Stahl, R.N.

*Ruthie Bernard, R.N.

Sharon Jackson, R.N.

Sabrinia Autrey, R.N.

*Served on Planning Committee for our hospital research project.

Sharon Hoffert, R.N.

Judy Duncan, R.N.

Control Units

Julie Poules, R.N.

Veda Smith, R.N.

*Pat Huse, R.N.

Olga King, R.N.

Anna Cross, R.N.

Willie Younger, R.N.

Chuck Bickell, R.N.

George Troksa, R.N.

Special Units for Test – Retest Validation

Karen Schmelter Lewis, R.N.

June Steele, R.N.

Tessie Fermil, R.N.

Theresa Muehler, R.N.

Cathy Ostrowski, R.N.

Laurel Valentino, R.N.

The writing of our book has been a team effort from the beginning. We appreciate especially our Nursing Advisory Group who gave us invaluable input. These individuals were also members of the initial research project Planning Committee. The nurses involved were the following:

Jane Walker, R.N., Coordinator, Quality Assurance

Brenda Terrell, R.N., Director, Educational Resource Services

Becky Hertz, R.N., DRG Nurse Reviewer

Paula Curran, R.N., Administrative Director, Gerontology Services (formerly Director 3W2)

From the beginning, the University has offered considerable support and encouragement. Doris Blaney is indeed grateful to the University for its generous sabbatical policy. We wish to thank Dr. Elizabeth Grossman (located in Indianapolis), Dean of the university-wide School of Nursing, and the following individuals at Indiana University Northwest: Chancellor Peggy Gordon

*Served on Planning Committee for our hospital research project.

Elliott, Dean Lloyd Rowe (Academic Affairs), the faculty in the School of Nursing, Robert Moran, Jr. (Director of the Library) who expediated our working in the library, Timothy Sutherland (Assistant Librarian) who conducted an excellent literature search, Cynthia Boysen (our Phi Beta Kappa Senior baccalaureate nursing student, who had all but her dissertation done toward a doctorate in Clinical Psychology when she came into nursing. In a nursing independent study, she reviewed all of the literature in an exceptional way. She is a fine young woman with tremendous research potential.), and Jess McHenry (graduate student in business and economics).

Special acknowledgment is given to Catherine Tallos, principal secretary supreme, for her able assistance in preparing the manuscript.

Last, but certainly not least, we wish to gratefully acknowledge the outstanding support and assistance provided by Nancy Mullins, Editor, J. B. Lippincott Company, and her fine staff. We were able to work together in a challenging situation and complete the book on schedule.

Contents

COST-EFFECTIVE NURSING PRACTICE: Guidelines for Nurse Managers

· PART ONE
Motivational Factors
Necessary for Success

1
Revolution
in Health Care

THIS CHAPTER provides an overview of the changes that have occurred in the health care delivery system in recent years. The historical events that preceded the advent of the prospective payment system and how that system works are sketched briefly. The discussion moves to the cost of health care in monetary terms and costs in the United States are compared with those in other industrialized countries. Costs in the United States are much higher than in other countries and the question is whether or not health care will follow the same trend as the automobile, steel, and electronics industries and succumb to foreign competition. After an overall view, a micro view is presented giving the steps that one automobile company and one insurance company have instituted to reduce their respective costs. The hospitals and how they have been affected by the cost-reduction efforts is the next topic. The chapter ends with a discussion of why nursing must be concerned with costs in order to survive in the era of cost containment and cost reduction.

HEALTH COSTS OUT OF CONTROL

The decade of the 1980s has been mainly a time of tremendous upheaval in the health care industry. When President Reagan signed into law the Social Security Amendments of 1983, a new era was introduced in the delivery of health care in the United States. This signaled the advent of the prospective payment system and the use of diagnostic related groups (DRG) to determine how much the federal government would pay for illness. Although the new law only affected those on Medicare, it had a more far-reaching impact than merely determining the amount of money that the federal government would pay for medical and hospital costs for the elderly. Private insurers, big business, unions, those that provide health insurance, those who pay for health insurance, and those who use health insurance were all watching to see the response of the health care delivery system.

For several years the cost of health care had been increasing at an alarming rate. During the time of double-digit inflation health costs were not singled out for any special attention.

However, once the level of inflation started on a downward trend the high cost of health care attracted the attention of the federal government, large employers, unions, and other consumer groups. What was the problem, and why hadn't health costs stopped escalating in a manner similar to other costs?

Because health care has never been under the control of consumers it does not fit an economic model based on supply and demand.[1] In the absence of any competition the demand, the supply, and the charge for services were set dogmatically by physicians and hospital administrators. When the federal government declared that, regardless of income, health care was the public's right and then proceeded to allocate ever-increasing funds to ensure that right, demand rose despite rising prices. The principal reason that rising prices were ineffective in curbing demand was the fact that the consumer, the ultimate user of health care services, was not paying for this right. The costs were being paid by the insurance companies, who provided the coverage to the employees of business and industry, and the federal government, who paid for the services used by the people eligible for its programs.

EARLY COST CONTROL EFFORTS

The insurance companies responded by increasing the premium rates. The government's initial response began more than 15 years ago, when it instituted the Voluntary Effort in 1972. This was an appeal to hospitals to monitor themselves and make a significant endeavor toward cost containment. It was not as successful as had been planned and the government then passed the 223 Limitations that placed a limit on the reimbursement they would pay hospitals.[2] These new regulations did not sufficiently reduce the government's obligation to pay for health care costs and, therefore, the Tax Equity Fiscal Responsibility Act (TEFRA) was passed in October, 1982, followed in 1983 by the Social Security Amendments.

INTRODUCTION OF PROSPECTIVE PAYMENT

TEFRA eliminated or reduced many of the subsidies or reimbursements that the government would pay health care institutions. The Social Security Amendments of 1983 introduced prospective reimbursement by DRG. This latter concept was a dramatic change from the method that the government, or any other purchaser of health care, had paid for services. Prior to the use of DRGs, reimbursement was determined retrospectively, that is, after the services were actually performed, and depended on the length of stay, the medication given, and laboratory work ordered, to mention a few. With the advent of the DRG system prospective reimbursement was used (*i.e.*, it was determined before services were delivered). It was a flat fee and was based on which DRG was assigned to a patient.

There can be exceptions to the flat fee payment, such as when a patient has a greater length of stay or unusually higher care cost than the average that has been set for a particular DRG. Patients who fall into this category are termed *outliers:* They are either day outliers (exceeding average length of stay) or cost outliers (exceeding average cost of care). Hospitals may be reimbursed for outliers on a reasonable cost-plus basis. When this situation occurs, however, hospitals must complete the detailed paperwork required and then request a Medicare visit to review the patient's record. The government may or may not decide to pay for the additional costs, based on the particular circumstances.

Since the federal government is the largest consumer of health care services and pays 60% to 70% of the health care costs, it is easy to see why the implementation of the DRG prospective payment schedules has had such a dramatic impact on the health care delivery system. Other third party payers and purchasers of health services are investigating how they might use the system.

Another type of prospective reimbursement that should be mentioned is the per-diem system, which is a fixed amount paid for each day in the hospital. This is not related to specific services rendered or diagnosed illness. California's MediCal Program adopted this type of reimbursement schedule in 1983. All hospitals in the state, who were interested in caring for MediCal patients, were required to submit bids on a per-diem rate for any patient admitted, regardless of the diagnosis. Hospitals whose bids were in the $400 to $600 per-diem rate were awarded contracts. Reimbursement is calculated at the per-diem rate multiplied by the number of hospitalized days. The concept behind this approach is that when a patient is admitted to a hospital the costs are usually higher than the per-diem rate; however, as the patient recovers the costs drop below the contract rate, which enables the hospital not only to recover its losses but also to make a profit. The institution must be careful that it does not release a patient too soon and thus lose the revenue-enhancing days.[2]

This approach has generated a great deal of competition among hospitals in California for MediCal's business. Other health care benefit payers are now negotiating with hospitals in some of the western states regarding per-diem contract rates.

COMPARISON OF HEALTH CARE COSTS

The discussion thus far has referred generally to the high cost of health care in the United States and to some methods used in an attempt to lower these costs. Specifically, what does health care cost in terms of dollars and cents?

One method of examining the cost of health care is to ascertain how much is spent in the United States on a per-capita basis and to compare that amount with what other industrialized nations spend per capita. In 1985, the United States spent $1500; the sum for West Germany was $900; $800 was spent in France; $500 was spent in Japan; and $400 was spent per capita in Great Britain.[3] Stop for a moment and reflect on these figures.

The United States prides itself on having the most advanced medical education in the world, the best nursing education in the world, and the most advanced medical technology in the world. One could conclude none of these accomplishments contributes much to cost-effectiveness. The United States spends three times the amount of money on health care that Japan does for every man, woman, and child, and almost four times the amount spent in Great Britain, which has a long history of socialized medicine. Although many inadequacies accompany socialized medicine, one would have to admit that it is very cost-effective (an outcome that it is not supposed to possess). Cost-effectiveness is supposed to be one of the components of the fee-for-services practice of the United States. Obviously, this has not been a practice since the 1950s, before all the third party payers became involved.

The case of Japan bears closer scrutiny. Their costs are not only low compared to the United States, but their health statistics are also among the best in the world. They have, for example, the lowest infant mortality and the least number of deaths from heart disease, and they lose the fewest number of work days because of illness.[3] These data are impressive, considering that they emanate from a country that lay in ruins in 1945, devastated by two atomic bomb attacks, with its industry destroyed, its government in chaos, and its morale shattered. Are we, as nurses, about to lose our positions to an imported Japanese health care delivery system?

SOME LESSONS FROM BUSINESS

Most nurses would be skeptical that such a scenario could evolve in the United States. Consider what happened to American counterparts in the business world. Look, for example, at the steel, automobile, and electronics industries, to see where the United States conceded to foreign competition, specifically from

Japan. American management techniques were supposed to be the envy of the world (or so we were told). The graduate schools of business were turning out thousands of people with MBA degrees, who were equipped with the latest management techniques designed to maintain our leadership position for generations to come. The rest of the world sent their most intelligent students to our universities to learn from us and to obtain the vaunted MBA. What happened in this process? Nobody wanted what the United States had to sell: the products were too expensive, the quality of workmanship was poor; and the design was not what people wanted.

There has been, and still is, a great deal of speculation about what happened to America's leadership position within the industrialized nations of the world. Among the more prominent arguments about how we lost our competitive edge are the following: antibusiness government regulations and tax policies; excessive labor costs, which include health insurance; restrictive trade barriers of foreign countries that do not give American products access to their markets; the "dumping" of foreign goods, which is the illegal practice of selling at less than cost in order to capture a market and force American competition out of business. The list of reasons for our loss of leadership in the marketplace, or excuses if you will, is endless.

It is interesting to note that with a few exceptions (Lee Iacocca and H. Ross Perot probably being the most prominent), business executives tend mainly to put the blame everywhere but on their leadership and management ability. For the sake of argument, could it have been possible that in their rush to maximize the return on the investment to their stockholders, American executives forgot to reinvest for modernization; that they had no time to be concerned about quality control; and that they ignored the consumers' demand for more efficient products? There is a lingering suspicion that some executives have treated the original business of their corporations like an unwanted stepchild and have looked elsewhere to invest their profits because they believed their return would be greater. It made no difference that thousands of workers in their original companies would be unemployed and thus would not be part of the market for any product.

Support for this supposition was stated in a main article in *The Wall Street Journal.*[4]

This year, for the first time since Arthur Anderson & Co.'s biennial survey of auto executives began in 1979, the officials listed their own "management practices" first among the industry's problems. "That's very positive," says Peter C. Van Hull, the Arthur Anderson consultant who compiles the survey. "It's just like being an alcoholic: you can't solve the problem until you face it."

But Detroit's tendency to blame its troubles on others lingers on. In January, for example, Ford President Harold A. Poling called for stiffer restraints on Japanese — car imports — even though the restraints were instituted in 1981 to let Detroit get back on its feet and 1986 was Ford's most profitable year (p 1).[4]

What connection has this with health care and, more specifically, with nursing? The purpose is to make you, the nurse, take notice of what is happening in health care and what has happened to other segments of our economic base when they were faced with a similar challenge for better quality, lower costs, and more efficient services. The physicians and hospital administrators have had their opportunity to make health care affordable: Their record does not lead to optimism in pursuit of this worthy goal. Nurses, if they seize this opportunity, can make a major contribution to this goal by insisting on nursing solutions to nursing problems — by working smarter, not harder.

Although the Japanese health statistics and costs are impressive, there is also evidence to suggest that they can be explained partly by factors other than the health care system. Differences in diets, life-styles, and working situations explain to some extent the disparity between American and Japanese health statistics. There is even some indication the Japanese have been changing their diets and life-style to reflect a more western mode and, as a result, have been evidencing some of the same health problems seen in the United States.

COST CONTROL MEASURES AT TWO COMPANIES

Another indication of how expensive health care has become is reflected in the cost figures for one large corporation. In 1983, Ford Motor Company spent $742 million in providing health insurance for their American employees. That cost represented an increase of $250 million over the previous 5 years. Health insurance added $300 to the cost of every Ford car produced in the United States.[5]

In an effort to contain rising costs Ford Motor Company initiated a strategy of promoting alternative health care programs. The company was trying to shift services away from expensive hospital care to appropriate lower cost settings and to stimulate competition among health care providers. In 1984, there was a total of 49 HMOs that Ford employees could elect to join in various locations throughout the country. The company estimated that it saved $7 million on insurance premiums alone through the enrollment of 8.7% of their eligible employees in HMOs. Ford Motor Company has also begun to use the services of preferred provider organizations (PPO) as another alternative.

It is not only the government and the business corporations that are trying to limit the high cost of health care. A major health insurance company has announced guidelines that would curb reimbursement for the 15 most common categories of diagnostic tests. On April 3, 1987, the Blue Cross and Blue Shield Association publicized their guidelines at the annual meeting of the American College of Physicians. The cost-reducing plan has drawn severe criticism from the College of American Pathologists, which states that the plan eliminates many tests for detecting health problems that are not immediately suspected by physicians. The pathologists were one of several medical groups consulted during the previous 3 years by Blue Cross and Blue Shield Association as it prepared the guidelines. Other medical organizations that support the plan are the American Society of Anesthesiologists, the American Thoracic Society, and the American Academy of Pediatrics.[6]

The annual savings from the guidelines are estimated to be from $6 billion to $18 billion nationally. The president of Blue Cross and Blue Shield stated that they spend about $27 billion a year on laboratory tests, $2 billion on chest roentgenograms, and another $1 billion on electrocardiograms, which amounts to 7% of their total expenditures for health care insurance claims. The president continued to say they estimated that 20% to 60% of these tests were unnecessary. Accordingly, the guidelines state that unless a patient has symptoms or a history of heart and chest disease they should not have chest roentgenograms or electrocardiograms as routine procedures. Blood cultures, complete blood counts, arterial blood gas analysis, throat cultures, and syphilis tests are also included in the category of routine tests that will be limited under the guidelines. The insurer plans to phase in the guidelines over the next year through physician education programs and scientific papers in the *Annals of Internal Medicine* (p 1).[7] Other health insurance companies are expected to support the guidelines and to move in a similar direction.

HEALTH COST AND THE GROSS NATIONAL PRODUCT

From the foregoing discussion it is apparent that major efforts have been expended to curb the ever-increasing costs of health care. These sanctions have not been very successful, according to a report from the Department of Health and Human Services. During 1985, the United States spent $425 billion on health care, which amounted to 10.7% of the gross national product (GNP), the highest share in history. This increase was 8.9% above 1984, and it was the lowest annual rate of increase in two decades. However, even that low increase in spending was far greater than the general rate of inflation that was 3.9% and the growth in the GNP of 5.6%. The report warned that health care inflation has not been brought under control and that outlays could continue to grow as a percentage of GNP.[8] The Department of Commerce estimates that by the end of 1987, health care expenditures will be $511 billion, which will represent 11.4% of the GNP.[9] The figures for 1986 indicate that the cost of health care grew seven times faster than the rate of general inflation. The Consumer Price Index (CPI) rose at 1.1%, whereas health care showed a 7.7% increase. Prescription drugs led the way with a 9% increase followed by an increase of 7.8% in doctors' fees, 7.7% in hospital room rates, and 5.5% in dentists' fees.[10]

These figures are not encouraging for bringing costs of health care lower or more in line with the general level of inflation. The pressure for cost containment will continue to be exerted on all members of the health care delivery system. This indicates that the old methods of providing health care will be outmoded: no more business as usual. Hospitals in particular have experienced a change in the use of their services. Nurses, as major contributors to hospital effectiveness, should be aware of and should be able to respond positively to the trends and problems confronting their primary source of livelihood.

EFFECT OF COST CONTROLS ON HOSPITALS

What are some of the other major trends that have impacted on hospitals? Nationally, inpatient care has not been emphasized as much, which has resulted in a decline in hospital admissions. In 1984, admissions declined 4% and in 1985, the decrease was 4.6%. Although some hospitals did not experience a decline in admissions, which reflected variations in local conditions, the downward trend was generally consistent across geographic regions, bed-sized groups, and various types of ownership. The steepest declines in admissions have tended to be among small hospitals, rural hospitals, and nonteaching hospitals. For the smallest bed-sized group (those with less than 25 beds), admissions fell 17.6% in 1985. However, for those hospitals having 500 or more beds, the decline was only 2.6%.[11] More recent data from hospitals suggest that the decline in admissions has slowed at the national level and in most regions and bed-sized groups. Admissions for the second quarter of 1986, dropped at less than half the rate of the previous year, −2.2% as compared to the second quarter of 1985, a −5.7% drop in admissions. Although the drop in admissions may be declining more slowly, economists with the American Hospital Association expect some decline to continue. This is the natural by-product of the growth in payment systems that discourages inpatient treatment. This moderation, however, of the decline in the admission rate may indicate that such controls could be approaching the point of diminishing returns.[12]

In addition to the reduction in hospital admissions there has also been a decline in a patient's length of stay in a hospital. For the 10-year period, 1975 to 1985, the average length of stay went from 7.7 days to 6.5 days.[13] This trend, however, also appears to be moderating. Nationally, in 1984, the length of stay dropped sharply for the groups of patients under age 65 and also over age 65. In the former group the drop was 3.6% and for the latter group the drop was 7.6%. There was a dramatic change in 1985:

The decline for those under age 65 was only 1.2% and for the group over 65 years of age, the decline was 2%. This leveling off was manifested in all regions of the United States and in all bed-sized hospitals.[11]

Moreover, in the first half of 1986, an even more interesting phenomenon occurred. A patient's average length of stay in hospital increased. Regardless of all the controls and incentives for an early discharge, the average length of stay grew 0.2%, which contrasted sharply with a 2.6% decline in the first half of 1985. These figures were gathered nationally from all bed-sized hospitals and all age groups. In an atmosphere that encourages outpatient care, the natural consequence of such a policy is that inpatients will be more severely ill. Given that scenario, the admitted patient will generally require a longer recovery time; hence the increase in average length of stay.[12]

A natural corollary of the decline in hospital admissions would be an increase in the number of outpatient visits. Since 1983, annual outpatient visits have risen by 14 million. A large increase came in 1985 with an increase of 4.8%, or nearly 11 million, compared to a 1.1% increase in 1984.[11] Through the third quarter of 1986 outpatient visits rose 8.3%, which was more than twice the 4.1% increase for the same period in 1985.[14] Although outpatient visits show no signs of moderation, it is also probably fair to assume that this sector of health care delivery will not continue to grow at such dramatic rates on a long-term basis. It is a natural progression for many new services to show impressive gains in utilization, after their initial acceptance as viable alternatives to establish methodology, and then to level off as the saturation point is reached. Setting limits on reimbursements for the delivery of health care provides a strong impetus for decisions to use new or different modes of treatments. As experience with outpatient services grows, however, it will be possible to make more reliable comparisons regarding cost-effectiveness and quality care between the inpatient and outpatient modality. In some cases it may be more efficient and less expensive to diagnose and care for the patient in the hospital, rather than in the clinic, which could then require additional costly care in the home.

Hospitals have been the recipients of most of the cost-cutting demands from the federal government and corporations. The results of these pressures have meant that, in many instances, hospitals have changed their method of operation: They have reduced traditional services and expanded into new services; they have joined other hospitals in voluntary associations and in other instances have been merged into multisystems; they have formed alliances and affiliations with HMOs, PPOs, and nursing homes. All of these actions, and others not listed, have been done for the purpose of survival. A survey by Touche Ross and Company, New York, of 1224 hospital administrators revealed that 43% feared that their facilities will close in the next 5 years.[15]

The possibility of so many hospitals closing is a very real fear, but hospital closings had been occurring long before the recent enactment of federal policies and corporate cost controls. Between 1976 and 1980 in New York City alone, 29 hospitals were closed and by 1982, another 17 were considered in financial distress. For the 5-year period, 1975 to 1980, the American Hospital Association (AHA) recorded a net loss of 186 hospitals, which was before the Reagan administration's health budget cutbacks. In1981, AHA reported that the total number of hospitals declined to 6933, which represented a loss of 33 hospitals and 3000 beds from 1980. These figures suggest that the closings were in smaller hospitals with 100 beds or less. Nationally in 1982, according to the Department of Health and Human Services, 160 hospitals were classified as being in financial distress in addition to the 17 hospitals in New York City, which have already been mentioned. An article in *The Wall Street Journal* on December 29, 1982 predicted that by 1990 about 1000 hospitals would be forced to close because of the money crunch.[16]

NURSING AND COST CONCERNS

While those earlier closings probably represented some adjustments to the building boom of the late 1950s through the 1960s and to the continued use of outmoded facilities, the closings that have been forecasted will be the result of inefficiencies and mismanagement. It is thus important for nurses to be aware of cost-effective nursing practices. For various reasons, which are discussed in this book, nurses have not felt compelled to be concerned about controlling costs. If nurses are not concerned about jobs or income or providing care to the ill, then they need not concern themselves with cost containment or cost reduction. If, however, they are concerned about jobs, and income, and providing care, then they must also become concerned about cost control.[3]

According to Stevens in the not-too-distant past when other health professionals were also not concerned with costs, nursing developed its own form of "unlimited resources" philosophy.[17] This philosophy has also been called total nursing care, total patient care, and comprehensive nursing care. It is a philosophy that appeals to the altruistic nature of nurses, the basic tenet being that regardless of cost, each patient deserves and should receive the best nursing care. Circumstances and the economy have changed, but nursing continues to cling to the same philosophy. Nursing students who are presently graduating are still taught that it is not professional and that it represents a failure on their part to provide anything less than comprehensive care. This enduring belief in comprehensive care could be a real threat to the continued existence of nursing in its present form. Such a philosophy, however laudable, will have difficulty working today. No additional resources are likely to be allocated to health care in the future; in fact, as has been emphasized earlier, the reverse is true. Cost containment and cost reduction are the goals of all purchasers of health care. In a world with finite resources, a philosophy for nursing must be compatible with reality. Nursing will either develop such a philosophy, or it will risk being replaced by other groups who are willing to respond to the challenge.[17] After all, to paraphrase a well-known cartoon character, 15 years from now, nursing does not want to be in the position of saying, "We have seen the enemy and it is us."

It is not the purpose of this book to develop a new or different philosophy of nursing. That exercise, however appealing, should be the topic of another work. Rather, in following the chapters the authors highlight nursing's pivotal position in the health care delivery system; direct attention to the power that nurses possess and how they can enhance it through assertiveness; offer research proven techniques to help nurses become more cost-effective in their performance; and offer a prognosis of future health care delivery and the role of nursing. The emphasis is on nursing solutions to nursing problems and on helping nurses to work smarter, not harder.

Questions for Reflection and Discussion

1. Why didn't rising prices curb the demand for health care?

2. How does prospective reimbursement differ from retrospective reimbursement, and which method does the federal government presently use?

3. What can cause exceptions to the flat fee payment schedule? Have any been used in your hospital?

4. Would you favor a per-diem reimbursement system instead of the DRG system? Explain why you think it would or would not work in your hospital?

5. From a personal standpoint, based on your experience, do you feel that the average hospital patient receives care commensurate with what his insurance pays for?

6. Do you believe a foreign group could successfully offer health care in the United States? Elaborate on your thinking and give the rationale for your decision.

7. Fifteen years ago, did you think the automobile, steel, and electronic manufacturing industries in the United States would be faced with their present competitive situation?

8. Do you believe that the managers in your hospital have the raison d'être of the hospital as their goal?

9. How do you view the action taken by Blue Cross and Blue Shield to curb the reimbursement of the 15 most common diagnostic tests?

10. How has the prospective payment system affected your hospital's admissions, patient's length of stay, and out-patient procedures?

11. Is it important for all nurses to understand how DRGs impact on your hospital?

12. Do you think your hospital is among the group that will close in the next 5 years? Give your reasons as objectively as possible.

13. If your hospital is a candidate for closing, what steps do you believe should be taken to prevent such an occurrence or should it be prevented?

14. Do you agree with Stephens that nursing needs a new philosophy of care. Consider it carefully in terms of both quality and cost-effective care.

REFERENCES

1. Lauver EB: Where will the money go? Economic forecasting and nursing's future. Nursing & Health Care 6:133, 1985
2. Strasen L: Key Business Skills for Nurse Managers. Philadelphia, JB Lippincott, 1987
3. Curtin L: A piece of the action. J Emerg Nurs 12:110, 1986
4. Ingrassia P, Naj AK: U.S. auto makers get chance to regain sales from foreign rivals. But will they blow it again? The Wall Street Journal April 16, 1987
5. Shelton J: Can nursing options cut health care's bottom line? Nursing & Health Care 5:251, 1984
6. James FE: Blue Cross plans coverage limits on many tests. The Wall Street Journal April 1, 1987
7. Blues to curb payments for routine tests. Health Care Competition Week April 6, 1987
8. Health-care spending's share of GNP reaches a new high. Medical Benefits, The Medical-Economic Digest August 31, 1986
9. Ginzberg E: New economic climate breeds new markets. Nursing & Health Care 8:139, 1987
10. Medical care costs grow seven times faster than inflation in 1986, p 1. Health Professions Report February 23, 1987
11. 1985 in review, admissions, outpatient visits, and length of stay. Economic Trends 1(5):2, 1986
12. Utilization declines level off, pp 1, 8. Aspen's Advisor For Nurse Executives December, 1986
13. Hospital discharges fall below 150 per 1,000, p 5. Washington Actions on Health October 13, 1986
14. Economics. Hospitals 61(3):34, 1987
15. Nursing's compelling agenda, p 1. Executive Director Wire Sept/Oct, 1986
16. Salmon JW: Profit and health care: Trends in corporatization and propriertization. Int J Health Services 15(3):395, 1985
17. Stevens BJ: Tackling a changing society head on. Nursing & Health Care 6:27, 1985

2
Conceptual Model of Nursing's Pivotal Position: Is the Nurse Prepared?

THE CASE manager will play a key role in the future of patient care delivery. Professional nurses, by virtue of their unique position in the patient care process, are ideally suited to fill this role. As the case managers of patient care, nurses in the hospital setting are with the patients 24 hours/day, 7 days/week, 52 weeks/year. They are the critical network link to quality and the continuity of care. Since they are managers of patient care, they have to be responsible and accountable not only for quality care, but also for cost-effective care; consequently, efforts to improve efficiency and control costs must necessarily include nurses.

Unfortunately, many nurses are ill-equipped to handle the demands and requirements of emerging cost-effectiveness programs and strategies. In the past, cost considerations were rarely an issue in providing quality patient care and most nurses received little or no systematic exposure or formal education in cost concepts or cost-effective nursing. Perhaps more problematic is the pervasive perception among nurses that a concern with cost-effective practices will inevitably result in lower quality patient care. Many nurses thus have a relatively uninformed and less-than-positive attitude toward cost-effectiveness.

The purpose of this chapter is to discuss a model of what the nurse's central role should be in patient care, both in the processing and management of the care. Some changes, challenges, and opportunities for nurses in this central role are addressed; critical training needs are assessed; and a responsive continuing education program is described.

NURSING'S PIVOTAL POSITION

A conceptual model of nursing's pivotal position has been developed in Figure 2-1. Within the model, nurses unquestionably

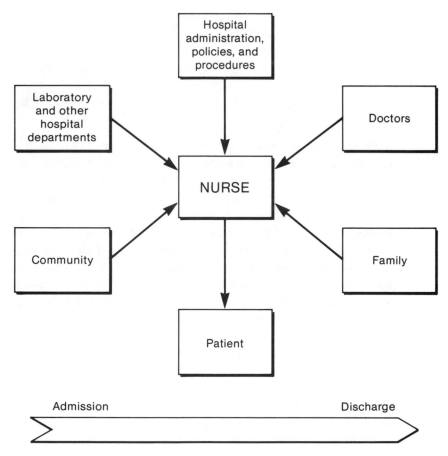

FIGURE 2-1. *Model of the nurse's central role in patient care, processing, and management. (Blaney/Hobson model © 1986)*

perform an indispensable role in managing patient care and in influencing their progress to discharge. The focal position occupied by nurses in relation to the hospital administration, laboratory and other departments, physicians, community, and the patient's family is shown in Figure 2-1. This model offers several challenges and opportunities for nurses to assume a leadership role as patient care managers from admission to discharge in developing and implementing cost-effective nursing practices and procedures.

STATE OF THE ARTS

Nursing is both a professional service and a holistic service. This statement is underscored by two facts: (1) discretionary judgment is required of professionals in their work, and (2) large amounts of data that do not always fit the model of exact science are required in order to make decisions concerning clinical practice.[1] The nurse is the central coordinator, the one person who interfaces with the physician, other hospital departments, patient, family, and community. The nurse is the only one who knows completely about the condition of the patient. The following examples highlight this fact.

Example 1

A diabetic patient is scheduled for foot surgery the next day. The podiatrist's primary concern is the surgery, not that the patient has diabetes. The nurse must coordinate the surgery for the patient by questioning IVs, insulin, and dietary orders, to mention a few.

Example 2

A patient received multiple units of blood and the calcium level began dropping. The nurse involved was aware of the numbers of transfusions and indicated this fact to the physician as a possible source for the low calcium.

Example 3

The family wanted no code blue papers signed for a terminal patient but the physician refused to sign them. It became the nurse's responsibility to bring the family and physician together to get the papers signed.

These examples show how nursing control facilitates the effective and efficient processing of the patient.

Nurses are all too familiar with examples of how control from outside nursing has caused problems in the delivery of care. The following examples are representative of the more common problems.

Example 1

A patient does not meet Utilization Review criteria and has to be discharged even though the nurses do not think that the patient is ready to be discharged, because more teaching (*i.e.*, colostomy care) is necessary. The patient will probably be readmitted to the hospital, which will prove more costly in the long run.

Example 2

A patient goes to a diagnostic department for tests and that department sends the patient directly to another department for further tests instead of back to the unit. Medications and treatments are therefore disrupted.

Example 3

Social Services makes decisions on discharge planning that might not be based on the patient's complete medical status.

Example 4

Other departments are not open on weekends, thus appropriate therapies and tests may be delayed.

Example 5

Housekeeping delays in cleaning rooms may necessitate placing patients in other units or may cause the patient to spend a long time in the Emergency Department waiting for a bed.

In summary, these examples indicate considerable fragmentation in scheduling. If these situations were controlled by the nurse, optimal scheduling of the patient could be coordinated efficiently and effectively and could help motivate the patient to an earlier discharge from the hospital.

CHANGE—OPPRESSED MINORITY BEHAVIOR

In order for nurses to assume this pivotal position one of the major changes that they must make individually and collectively is to stop behaving as an oppressed group. Roberts contends that nurses have characteristics such as other oppressed groups which,

> ". . . stem from the ability of dominant groups to identify their norms and values as the 'right' ones in the society and from their initial power to enforce them. In most cases of oppression, the dominant group looks and acts differently from the subordinate group (*i.e.*, black versus white, men versus women), and the characteristics of the subordinate group becomes negatively valued."[2]

Roberts states that nurses are oppressed because they do not really control their profession.[2] Instead, many physicians and hospitals exploit nurses and have benefited by controlling them. As a result nurses display "horizontal violence" where they act out against each other and do not support one another, because they feel unable to attack the oppressor.

The oppressed nurses display various fears of destruction by the dominant group; of change itself; and of success.

In order for the oppressed groups to be liberated, Freire describes two necessary requirements: (1) unveiling of the world of oppression, and (2) expulsion of the myths created and developed by the old order.[3] It is critical to freedom that the oppressed function autonomously and develop a sense of pride. Freire states that "Freedom is acquired by conquest not by gift."[3] Autonomy is not granted by the oppressor, instead it must be acquired by the oppressed. To make the change it is important to know about the concept of oppression so that the group understands thoroughly the factors involved. It is equally important that the leaders who can have a positive impact on the group and change the oppressed behavior must come from the expanded group. The leader should not come from the elite and should not be someone who has more loyalty to the oppressor. The result will be the development of unity and pride. For this successful leadership to occur, the leader must be involved continuously and must communicate with all the members of the group.[3]

LeRoux recommends, "one of our tasks in nursing is to motivate nurses not only to imagine the unimagined but also to become aware of how their social conditioning has affected them."[4]

Nurses must stop being so tough on each other and they must learn to trust and support one another. Only through a united effort can nurses assume leadership roles and exert influence. With the advent of DRGs and the government moving from a retroactive to a prospective payment mode for Medicare patients (as noted in the previous chapter), a revolution in the health care industry has occurred. Professional nurses need not fear this revolution because several challenges and opportunities exist.

CHALLENGES AND OPPORTUNITIES

This is a wonderful opportunity to demonstrate what is involved in professional nursing. Nurses have the opportunity to demonstrate their real value. They can show the difference that their time makes in changing the patient's condition.

Clinical and financial data are being brought more closely together. At last, the goal of the nurse and the hospital is the same — to get the patient out of the hospital as soon as possible with the best care possible. Nurses must focus on the relationship between practice and the hospital. What are the values of the hospital? No values should be more important than quality service. There are necessary changes in the primary focus from cure to care. The care values are that the patient deserves the best resources possible and the nurses are the best people to develop and manage these services.

Cost, which is a large problem, can be controlled by professional nurses. The cost of care was never previously an issue for nurses. They are now becoming and have to become more conscious of costs and, therefore, more productive in allocating nursing resources.

One of the results of a study conducted by Sovie and associates at Strong Memorial Hospital (SMH) and a Community Hospital in Rochester, New York was as follows.[5]

When DRG's with only a limited number of patients are removed from the analysis, the average direct nursing costs within average total room costs fall within a range of 18 to 24%. This is with a predominantly RN staff, and challenges the belief that such a staffing mix is expensive. With a 92% RN staff, for example, the average nursing care hours for DRG 121 were 70 at SMH and 125 in a neighboring Rochester community hospital, that reported a staff mix of 52% RN's; for DRG 122 it was 56 hours for our hospital and 90 hours for the other (Table 2-1).[5]

Good care by professional nurses can shorten the patient's stay in hospital. The professional nurses know that people are the most important asset in the hospital. On a particular unit in regard to the productivity of the unit, they each know they are only as good as the other professional nurses with whom they collaborate on a daily basis. Each nurse is in a pivotal position to control costs.

The nursing department must be the competitive edge for the hospital's public relations on a 24-hour basis — a vital link between quality and cost, because this department is responsible for the continuous care of the patient. In this regard, nurses will advance in a meaningful way when they realize that they can make an important and valuable contribution, and when they respect themselves as professionals who hold the key position in quality, cost-effective patient care.

Nurses are in the upper 10% of the population in intelligence. Top performers do significantly better than the norm. Mediocrity should not be tolerated. A real challenge is to recognize this fact and help these nurses change their attitudes and behaviors. Efficiency should be rewarded.

Nurses must develop a marketing plan for the services that they offer to the community (*i.e.*, by visibility). They must understand thoroughly how valuable the patient contact is in such a marketing approach. As competition increases, patients will be drawn by the quality of care.

In marketing, the concept of selling is not the only one to consider. Nurses should make people feel welcome by reassuring anxious parents and by helping people who need their services. These services involve competence, caring, compassion, and at the same time, competition.

Professional nurses can become cost-effective managers. They know that nursing is necessary for individuals. They can learn that they must both monitor productivity and defend the budget.

Table 2-1. Comparison of Selected Strong Memorial Hospital and Rochester Hospital Findings for Two Diagnostic Related Groups

Diagnostic Related Groups	Strong Memorial Hospital			Rochester Community Hospital		
	No. Patients	Average Nursing Hours	Average Direct Nursing Costs	No. Patients	Average Nursing Hours	Average Direct Nursing Costs
121 AMI with CV Compl Disch Alive	91	69.59	$752	16	125	$1065.00
122 AMI without CV Compl Disch Alive	211	56.58	$611	19	90	$ 766.80

AMI = anterior myocardial infarction; CV Compl = cardiovascular complications; Disch = discharge.

(Sovie MD, Tarcinale MA, VanPutte AW, Stunden AE: A Correlation Study of Nursing Patient Classification, DRGs, Other Significant Patient Variables, and Cost of Patient Care. Unpublished study report. Rochester, NY, University of Rochester, 1984; Lagona TG, Stritzel MM: Nursing care requirements as measured by DRG. J Nurs Admin 14(5):15–18, 1984.)

COST-EFFECTIVENESS CAN BE TAUGHT

There is a simple formula in psychology regarding performance.

Performance = ability × motivation

This formula suggests that cost-effectiveness can be taught.

We conducted research from February 1984 to June 1985 regarding attitudes and behaviors concerning cost-effective nursing practices.[6]

In a medium-sized midwestern hospital, a seven-person advisory committee — consisting of nurses, nurse supervisors, and key nurse administrators — collaborated with nursing and business faculty to develop a seven-hour nurse training program on cutting costs. This group both identified major problem areas and suggested potential solutions.

The program consisted of, first, a general discussion of the principles of the nurse's power and influence in the hospital. This was followed by an overview of the new financial and competitive pressures being exerted on modern hospitals and the critical need for greater cost efficiency.

The overriding personal relevance of this issue to each nurse was emphasized. The industrial- and professional-service models of product management were compared.

Next, strategies were presented to address the three major problem areas identified by the advisory committee. Specific procedures designed to improve awareness of supply costs and enhance efficient use were presented. Goal setting as an approach to motivate timely patient recovery was then discussed. Finally, the critical-path method of production scheduling was introduced as a model to aid optimal scheduling of tests and procedures.

In all instances, experiential exercises and actual hospital cases were used to illustrate each new procedure and allow for hands-on participant interaction and practice. The session concluded with the discussion of major changes, challenges, and opportunities facing nursing.

Subjects. Eight nursing units participated in the study: four units in the experimental group (to receive the training), four in the control group (not to receive the training). Nursing units were matched in terms of size and patient mix. A total of 156 nurses participated in the study — 78 in the experimental group, 78 in the control group.

Results. Several criteria were measured. One was the nurse's job performance on the three critical issues identified by the nursing advisory committee: supply use, patient training and motivation, and patient scheduling.

Head nurses in both the experimental and control groups evaluated the staff on the three dimensions, first before training and then afterward.

Scores on the three dimensions were summed to provide a composite index of cost-effective performance for each nurse, with scores ranging from a low of 3 to a high of 27. Higher scores indicated more cost-effective performance.

The experimental group's mean performance score of 15.30 after the training was significantly higher than its pretraining mean of 11.23 (t = 8.89, df = 68, P < .001); its score was also higher than the control group's mean score of 11.28 (t = 5.06, df = 146, P < .001).

In the first full month after the training program, the mean length of patient stay in the experimental group was 11 percent lower than the mean in the control group.

Moreover, the mean length of patient stay in the first full month after the training program was 17 percent lower on the experimental units than those units' similar mean in the same month one year earlier.

On yet another criterion — nonsalary unit operating costs, including nonbillable drugs, supplies, minor equipment, and miscellaneous items — cost-saving awareness and strategies made a difference.

During the first full month after the training program, the mean nonsalary operating cost in the experimental group was 22 percent lower than the comparable figure in the control group. The experimental units also had a 3 percent lower mean nonsalary operating cost in the first full month after the training than their mean for the same month one year earlier (p 187).[6]*

Can cost-effectiveness be taught? For professional nurses to hold the pivotal role in the delivery of quality cost-effective care, we have no doubts, based on our research, that it can and must be taught.

IS THE NURSE PREPARED?

The first section of the book identifies and discusses motivational factors necessary for successful and cost-effective nursing performance. These include enhancing nursing power and self-

*From Hobson CJ, Blaney DR: Techniques that cut costs, not care. Am J Nurs 87(2):185, 1987. © American Journal of Nursing Company.

confidence, proper attitudes, incentives, and performance appraisal systems.

The second section describes ability factors necessary for success. They include the following necessary knowledge and skills: cost controls, efficient use of supplies, optimal scheduling, goal setting to motivate the patient to early discharge, managing time effectively, and physical fitness for the nurse to improve productivity.

The two central themes of the book for the reader to keep in mind are (1) nursing-based solutions to nursing problems, and (2) working smarter, not harder!

Information in this book can be an investment. There are many ideas that will allow the nurse to provide better patient care in a more cost-effective manner. Each nurse will gain the wisdom of knowing that she can make a difference in cost-effective nursing practices.

Questions for Reflection and Discussion

1. Do you believe that nurses hold a pivotal role in patient care processing and management? Do you believe that they are prepared adequately for this role?

2. In the conceptual model six groups have been identified with which the nurse coordinates care: hospital administration, physicians, family, laboratory and other hospital departments, community, and patient. Can you identify other key groups that should be included in the model?

3. Why should nursing control the patient care process?

4. Are there other groups in the health care delivery process that should play the controlling, pivotal role? Why would these groups fail to do it as well as nurses?

5. Some examples are given concerning how nursing control facilitates the effective and efficient processing of the patient. Identify other examples. How many nurses understand clearly the importance of this control?

6. Examples were given regarding how control from sources other than nursing has caused problems in the delivery of patient care. Identify other examples. What could nurses do to eliminate these problems?

7. Develop a protocol on each shift which focuses on the behavior with which nurses are involved concerning the public relations of the hospital. Who would you give these protocols to?

8. Develop a marketing plan for your unit. Operationalize the concepts of competence, caring, compassion, and competition as they relate to cost-effective patient care. How would you implement this plan?

9. Identify three fears that oppressed groups exhibit. What type of leaders can impact positively on the oppressed? Should the head nurse fill this role?

10. What are three tried-and true methods of cutting costs by 20% without compromising care? How can you use these techniques in your work?

REFERENCES

1. Hegyvary ST: Perspectives on Nursing Productivity. In Davis A, Levine E (eds): The National Invitational Conference on Nursing Productivity, April 16–18, 1986, Proceedings. Georgetown University Hospital Nursing Department and Georgetown University School of Nursing, p 88
2. Roberts J: Oppressed group behavior: Implications for nursing. Adv Nurs Sci 5(4):21, 1983
3. Freire P: Pedagogy of the Oppressed, p 31. New York, Herder and Herder, 1971
4. LeRoux R: Power, powerlessness, and potential—nurse's role within the health care delivery system. Image 10(3):26, 1978
5. Sovie MD: A correlation study of nursing patient classification, DRG's, other significant patient variables and cost of patient care. In Davis A, Levine E (eds): The National Invitational Conference on Nursing Productivity, April 16–18, 1986, Proceedings. Georgetown University Hospital Nursing Department and Georgetown University School of Nursing, p 48
6. Hobson CJ, Blaney DR: Techniques that cut costs, not care. Am J Nurs 87(2):185, 1987

Enhancing Nursing Power, Self-Perceptions, and Assertiveness

AS A nurse, how powerful do you feel? How much power do you actually have in your work place, in your practice, and as a person? In the next decade it will be crucial for the profession of nursing and for the delivery of quality, cost-effective nursing practice that nurses become powerholders in all three areas.

The purpose of this chapter is to discuss six aspects of power: (1) to introduce the nurse to the importance of power, (2) to define power and review the various models of power, (3) to introduce a newly developed integrated model of power within the context of cost-effective nursing practices, (4) to discuss the types of power, (5) to describe the dimensions of power, and (6) to provide an exercise for nurses to develop their self-awareness and self-esteem in order to become powerholders.

IMPORTANCE OF POWER

Although nurses may not admit to it, they have always had power. The visionary founder of modern nursing, Florence Nightingale, exemplified power. The evidence of one major change, brought about through her powerful leadership, is recorded in history. During the Crimean War, the death rate of the soldiers dropped dramatically from 427:1000 (42%) to 22:1000 (2.2%) over 6 months after only 38 self-proclaimed nurses arrived in Scutari. An estimated three quarters of the soldiers who were casualties were not dying in battle, but from dysentery, cholera, typhoid, and infection, which they had contracted in the hospital. The nursing care given by those few nurses and the changes made in the delivery of care made the dramatic difference in the death rate in a short time.[1] This was power!

Nurses are still powerful. They provide an essential service required by society. The social phenomenon of *need* generated power. The issue involved is the ways in which nurses have used, abused, and misused their power (or failed to use it at all) and the structure in which nursing has evolved and is now practiced.[2]

How powerful do nurses feel as providers of patient care and how do they perceive others in the hospital? Most nurses feel powerless to change the system. They believe that the administration has all the power and that nurses have none. Nurses *do* have power with their patients. They also have power within their unit; however, a great deal depends on the unit manager's power style. With respect to other departments, nurses feel that they lack power to influence patient care and to create changes within the departments.

Nurses in the decade of the 1990s must not only use the power that they have, but must also expand it. As the managers of patient care, nurses have not only to be responsible and accountable for quality care but also for cost-effective care. Nurses can no longer "bury their heads in the sand" and believe that someone else will worry about costs. This attitude leads to a mediocre performance that should not be tolerated. Efficiency will be rewarded. Top performers giving quality care can shorten the patient's stay in hospital. The goal of nursing and administration will be synchronized: This signifies considerable power for nurses. It is not an insurmountable task for nurses to achieve; like Florence Nightingale's success in Scutari, only a few nurses are required to initiate change.

DEFINITION AND MODELS OF POWER

Several definitions of power follow. Power, like love, is an emotional word that is used frequently and intuitively in ordinary language. The origin of the word *power* comes from the Latin verb *potere,* which means to be able.

Lasswell viewed power as an interpersonal situation and as a value.[3] He viewed the power seeker negatively by connecting the concept of power to personality theory. He regarded power as a compensatory means against deprivation. Consequently, a person with low self-esteem required help by the power-seeking person in order to raise his self-concept.[3]

From a sociological perspective, Mills[4] viewed power as residing in three major groups or institutions: the military, political, and economic elites; and, that "power resides along with wealth in and through these three major institutions." (p 9) "The Power Elite of our American society are composed of men whose positions in institutions enable them to transcend the ordinary men and women — they make the decisions that have major consequences for the rest of the society." (p 4)

Grissum and Spengler state that "in our society the individuals who control the purse strings, control others. They are the ones with recognized power" (p 51).[5] As noted above, Mills had a similar focus on money or economics as the procurer of power.[4]

Nurses must realize that for the first time their goal and the hospital's goal are synchronized (*i.e.,* to give the patient quality care and then facilitate discharge as quickly as possible). Nurses have the opportunity to seize the power and exert financial control by providing cost-effective nursing care. Will you, the nurse, exert the strength, energy, and action to become the powerholder in this endeavor?

Sociologist Hawley indicates that, "Every social act is an exercise of power, every social relationship is a power question, and every social system is an organization of power" (pp 422–431).[6] Some people regard power incorrectly like money, as an item that can accumulate. Power is not like this; instead, it is a relationship between two or more individuals. Furthermore, there is no certain amount allotted to one society. All power is relative. One person may have more power than a second person, but less power than a third. "The fact that one person possesses power does not mean that another person lacks power. Rather, persons possess degrees of power that vary with time and circumstances" (pp 2–4).[7] This elementary concept escapes most nurses; hence, their feelings of powerlessness.

Mechanic defines power as "any force that results in behavior that would not have occurred if the force had not been present" (p 351).[8] He regards power as more than a relationship; he views it as control over one's self first, then over information, persons, and institutions.

Berle, a close advisor to Presidents Franklin Roosevelt, Kennedy, and Johnson, addressed the concept of Power Form. "Coalescence of three elements — assertive men, an idea system, and a group capable of organization — generates power, be the measure small or great. It thereupon attains reality and assumes form. It has an impact on its environment" (p 55).[9] It thus achieves an image.

Craig and Craig define power as "the capacity of an initiator to increase his satisfaction by intentionally affecting the behavior of one or more responders" (p 45).[10] They discuss *synergistic power,* which brings together unlike factors to form a new product for action. Synergism is shared pursuit of independent individuals in which the sum effect of the joint action is greater than the total of the effects of each action taken independently. A synergistic leader has the capability to raise the satisfactions of all participants by deliberately bringing about increased energy and creativity to "co-create a more rewarding present and future" (p 62).[10]

The relationship of strength, energy, and action is seen by Claus and Bailey[11] as a pyramidal force, "with *strength* (the ability) as one of the elements supporting *energy* (the willingness to use the ability), which in turn supports the action itself" (p 17) (Fig. 3-1).

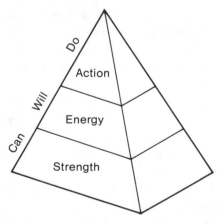

FIGURE 3-1. *The power pyramid. (Reproduced with permission from Claus K, Bailey I: Power and Influence in Health Care, p 18. St. Louis, CV Mosby, 1977)*

They consider their definition neutral for the following reasons: "(1) allows for the positive or negative use of power; (2) provides for the use of different types of power; (3) enables power to be used by persons, groups, or organizations; (4) is not tied to dependency relationships; and (5) focuses on results and use" (p 19).[11]

In analyzing these three basic components of power, Claus and Bailey emphasize the importance of *strength* (can) and they believe that without it an individual will not be powerful.[11] Ability and competence originate from strength. The individual who is strong concentrates on her strengths and either deemphasizes any weaknesses or tries to improve them. This is a powerful strategy. The *energy* (will) component follows. A strong person who is powerful has ample energy. This type of energy can be emitted readily to other individuals and can impact on their attitudes and behavior. In order to have a constant supply of energy, one must keep it operative in a continuous and uniform manner; otherwise, it may be lost — in other words, use it or lose it. *Action* (do), as the third component, is key to the powerful person. The goal of the powerful person is the ability to influence the performance of others. The powerholder, through the problem-solving and decision-making processes, releases motivational vigor inside others and stimulates them in goal-setting behaviors. The powerful person develops both personally and professionally as a result of this. "A powerful person grows in many dimensions: enhancing power, acquiring new authority, developing new skills, meeting new people, making new alliances, and striving for self-control. The powerful person deals in results. Power can be measured by results. When people are motivated to use positive forces of power within themselves one may observe differences in their behavior. A powerful person uses energy and strength to get things done and encourages and rewards cooperation and collaboration. Others want to do things for a powerful person" (pp 19–20).[11]

INTEGRATED MODEL OF POWER IN CONTEXT OF COST-EFFECTIVE NURSING PRACTICE

The Blaney/Hobson model of the nurse's central role in patient care, processing, and management is described in Chapter 2. Figure 3-2 illustrates how this model was modified and combined

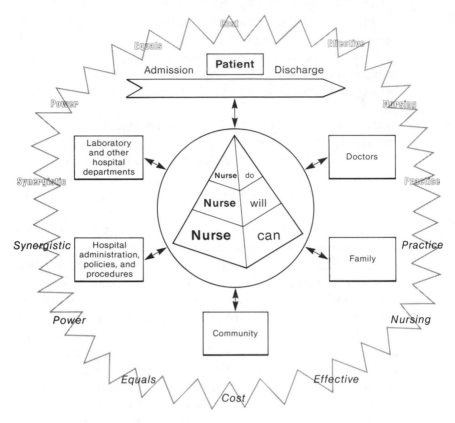

FIGURE 3-2. *Blaney/Hobson integrated model of power within the context of cost-effective nursing practice.*

with both the Claus and Bailey power pyramid, and Craig and Craig's concept of synergistic power into an integrated model of power within the context of cost-effective nursing practice.

Claus and Bailey's view of the model can give direction to nurses at all levels of practice.[11] It has a straight-forward message — CAN, WILL, and DO. With the emphasis on cost containment the nurse, as manager of patient care, is in an ideal position to implement cost-effective nursing practices. Since Florence Nightingale's time, nurses have had strength (both physical and mental) and abundant energy, and they have acted competently. However, for most nurses, this combination of ingredients has not been viewed from the perspective of a power-holder, able to consistently influence the performance of others through the manipulation of persons and organizations.

The Blaney/Hobson model is a dynamic interaction between the nurse as a powerholder and others, such as the hospital administration, laboratory and other hospital departments, physicians, families, and, most important, the patient. A nurse who is strong and energetic can play an important part in motivating the patient to an early discharge from the hospital. Radiating around this dynamic interaction is the synergistic power that Craig and Craig identified, which forms a new product for action by bringing together different constituents.[10] In this case the new product equals cost-effective nursing practices.

The biggest problem facing hospital administration — cost containment — can prove beneficial for nurses. Quality, cost-effective nursing practices can shorten the patient's stay in the hospital. The present is a wonderful occasion to demonstrate what professional nursing is all about, through powerful leadership.

In pursuing the concept that the capacity of power is to influence some aspect of the behavior of others, the powerful leader should consider the essential elements of power. Psychologist Jack Harsanyi[12] identifies seven aspects of the concept of power that merit examination within the context of the Blaney/Hobson integrated model of power as follows:

1. BASE of power: the resource or assets that a person can use to influence another

2. MEANS of power: the specific actions by which one can use resources (*i.e.*, threats and promises to influence behavior)

3. SCOPE of power: the set of specific actions that one person can get another to perform by using her means of power

4. AMOUNT of power: the net increase in the probability that someone will perform some specific action as the result of the use of power of one person over another

5. EXTENSION of power: the number of individuals over which the powerholder exercises control

6. COST of power: the opportunity costs of using power; more accurately, the costs of one's power over another is defined as the expected value (actuarial value) of the costs of one's attention to influence another

7. STRENGTH of power: the opportunity costs of the one on whom power is being exerted to resist the power

The sum of these aspects governs an individual's power in a particular context.

TYPES OF POWER

Unfortunately, numerous individuals, including nurses, feel that power is primarily a negative capacity. They function from a perspective of what sociologists call the "necessary evil" concept of power, dubbing it as "bad," "corrupting," or "dirty." The reality of the situation is that power is neither intrinsically good nor bad. A respected leader might be identified as having "good power" whereas a dominant figure from the crime syndicate who governs by coercion would be labeled as having "bad power." Power is an important part of every type of association, both on a personal basis as well as a professional one.

One of the most popular theories of power was developed by French and Raven.[13] They described five bases of power: reward, coercive, legitimate, referent, and expert.

The basis for *reward power* is the ability to provide a reward for desired behavior or change in behavior. Through effective use of the nursing process, especially focusing on goal setting to motivate the patient to be discharged early, nurses can give rewards by verbally reinforcing behaviors toward this end.

Coercive power, like reward power, involves manipulation; however, in this case the powerholder punishes the individual for undesired behavior. Unfortunately, nurses use this type of power too frequently; for example, withholding pain medication for a patient who is a whiner in order to "get even."

Legitimate power is the case where one individual has a legitimate right to dictate change in another's behavior because of the role of authority that she holds. In a decentralized nursing service organization, head nurses are in positions of legitimate power has been cited as a concern in nursing.[14] Although a large proportion of nursing students is from the upper one quarter of scheduling of procedures. It is essential for both the profession of nursing and the well-being of the patient that nurses use this type of power.

The basis for *referent power* is an individual's identification with or attractiveness to another. Wolf contends that this type of power has been cited as a concern in nursing.[14] Although a large proportion of nursing students is from the upper one quarter of their high school class, she laments, "One would never guess the intellectual capacities of nurses from their portrayal in books, movies, and television" (p 76).[14]

Both individual nurses and organized nursing groups have objected to these negative images; instead, they now emphasize the positive, more accurate role of the nurse through special media awards that are presented annually by the American Academy of Nursing.

Expert power comes from the idea that the more powerful individual has greater knowledge than the person who is less powerful. Wolf asserts, "Nursing is beginning to view itself as a learned profession with the need to know why, as well as the need to know how. The recognition of the existing levels of nursing practice with the identifications of separate roles and separate knowledge bases is another step toward expert power. The recognition of the independent nature of nursing practice with its inherent rights and responsibilities — including accountability — is another essential move toward expert power and control. The consumer must be able to recognize and request nursing services based on competent practice and knowledge. Nursing concomitantly, must be responsible for demonstrating its unique expertise in the health care system" (p 77).[14]

Nurses do have considerable expert power, but because of a lack of confidence and assertive behavior, they frequently succumb to the physician as the health provider with superior knowledge. As the case managers of patient care, nurses in the hospital setting are with the patients at all times during the year; in other words, they are the critical network link to quality and continuity of care. In these days of high competition that hospitals are faced with, and with most patients admitted to hospitals because they *need* nursing care, a nurse's expert knowledge can make the difference between whether a hospital survives or closes. That fact alone places the nurse in a powerful position.

Expert power, where one person does not have to be a member of a powerful person's group, is identified as *informational power*.[13] This type of power defers to an individual's proficiency to use explanations or other convincing statements to change the behaviors of others. A delegate at a convention who goes to the microphone and speaks eloquently concerning the advantages of a certain issue, then sways the delegation to vote for approval of a motion, is using informational power.

All of these different types of power bases are not mutually exclusive. A nurse must have all of these power bases to be an outstanding leader in nursing.

DIMENSIONS OF POWER

Women and Power

The nurse must ask herself if she wants to be a powerful leader. Nurses, who are predominantly female, have struggled with the traditional pattern of female role behavior. Kirkpatrick points out that "the pursuit of power (is) conceived as incompatible with femininity . . . Simultaneously, cultural norms communicate and reinforce the expectation of women's commitment to home, family, community service" (pp 14–15).[15]

The use of power is related to conventionally masculine traits. Male and female behavior, as studied by Petro and Putnam,[17] is compared in the box, Contrast of Commonly Held Behaviors Between Females and Males.

Kalish and Kalish give additional understanding into the cultural connection of men with power and women without power from a historical viewpoint.[7] "Men have been seen as strong, vigorous, competitive, and interested in money, power, and self-advancement. Women, on the other hand have been viewed as weak, soft, intuitive, compassionate, and interested in moral, humanitarian goals" (p 23).[7] Whereas women focus their attention on individuals, men are more concerned with financial gains. Competition, peer relationships that enhance hierarchical decision making, and complete domination over the formal and important manifestations of power have been the historical lot of humans. In contrast, the women stressed interpersonal relationships and cooperation that promoted a sharing, nonstructured decision-making manner. Women have had to depend on passive–aggressive behaviors whereas men display the complete opposite behaviors with assertiveness and aggression. Much of these differences have been the result of centuries of dominance of women by men, and the absence of any control in the political, social, and economic arenas.[7]

CONTRAST OF COMMONLY HELD BEHAVIORS BETWEEN FEMALES AND MALES

Male	Female
Realistic (not idealistic)	Unrealistic (idealistic)
Almost always hides emotions	Does not hide emotions
Always thinks before acting	Never thinks before acting
Not easily influenced	Easily influenced
Not excitable in crises	Excitable in crises
Active	Passive
Competitive	Not competitive
Feelings not easily hurt	Feelings easily hurt
Can make decisions easily	Difficulty making decisions
Never cries	Cries easily
Intellectual	Not intellectual
Good sense of humor	Poor sense of humor
Never worried	Always worried
Feels superior	Feels inferior
Doesn't care about being in a group	Greatly prefers being in a group
Seeks out new experiences	Avoids new experiences
Assertive	Not assertive
Unable to devote self completely to others	Able to devote self completely to others
Blunt	Tactful
Not kind	Kind
Not understanding of others	Understanding of others
Cold in relations to others	Warm in relations to others
Comfortable when people express emotions	Uncomfortable when people express emotions

(Petro CS, Putnam BA: Sex-role stereotypes: Issues of attitudinal changes. Sex Roles: A Journal of Research 5:33, 1979[16])

According to Kalish and Kalish, "Historically, women have assumed the role of wife and mother as their 'primary' role. Combining this role with a professional role has been viewed as incompatible, and trying to get a career launched in mid-life, after children are grown, is fraught with difficulties, given the competitive nature of our society" (pp 24–25).[7]

In an excellent paper presented at the Journal of Nursing Administration Conference, McClure coined the concepts of white-collar and blue-collar nurses.[17] Job-oriented nurses (blue-collar workers) focus primarily on the job and the earnings received from the actual work performed. They prefer structured settings and explicit job descriptions and usually work to contribute a second income in most family situations. They commonly display stereotype female behaviors as described in the box, Contrast of Commonly Held Behaviors Between Females and Males.

In contrast, career-oriented nurses (white-collar workers) have a life-long commitment to both the profession of nursing and education as a life-long process in which to strengthen their power bases. Although income is important it is not the primary motivator of performance. They are cognizant of the feminist issue of equal pay for comparable work, and they promote this cause.[18]

Smith states, "The career-oriented nurse, who may be characterized by attributes such as enthusiasm and assertiveness, needs to be challenged and rewarded. The job oriented nurse needs to be acknowledged for her contributions, but not placed in roles which require more than she can give. The job-oriented nurse is frequently content to do her job while 'on duty,' but makes a distinct delineation between being 'on duty,' and the remainder of her life. The notion of unification of one's being into a professional person does not exist for her. (This unification does not imply an inability to put aside the stresses of a job, but does imply that with a career-oriented nurse the total image and commitment to the profession is not a time-bound function.)" (pp 87–88).[18] Smith continues, ". . . believes the dilemma is a prominent example of the disparity which exists among women: the conflict of career-orientation versus job-orientation. The conflict for women is not so much between career and family, as between a real lifelong career versus limited participation in the work force" (p 88).[18]

Garant notes that in order to attain authority and become educated to practice, nurses have had to expend considerable energies.[19] "The struggle has been long and is far from being over—in fact, the battleground may have been determined only recently. Nursing, as a predominantly women's profession, has been (and is) struggling to gain and keep whatever power it can so that it can continue to exist" (p 192).[19] There is no consensus for nurses about wanting, getting, and retaining power: Some are attracted to power and all it stands for, and others are repulsed by the thought of it. The ambivalence mirrors the quandary: not to make a decision is to make a decision; or, desiring to be free from responsibility and accountability, and yet craving independence and autonomy.[19]

Interdependence and Power

Boyle emphasizes the importance of interdependence, which will assist all nurses in enhancing their power when they both understand their own expertise and the expertise of their colleagues.[20] By frequent collaboration involving discussions of knowledge, skills, and attitudes concerning the scope of their practice, nurses not only improve their practice, but also, the quality of care to patients. "Increasing the total amount of power in a situation by pooling individual power recognizes that the whole is greater than the sum of its parts" (p 165).[20]

An example of this situation involves the nurse–physician relationship. More experienced nurses who are self-confident and who have high self-esteem tend to be more effective with physicians and others. They are not only confident about their abilities but they can readily communicate their knowledge to physicians and others. When a physician knows and trusts a nurse's abilities, that nurse has more power with that physician. Nurses who lack power with a certain physician should seek a nurse who does to discuss patient care issues or requests. In the same manner, staff nurses might defer to a charge nurse or head nurse to intervene when dealing with other departments.

Another situation that occurs frequently in the hospital involves a nurse who is taking care of a demanding, manipulative patient and feels little power in dealing with this patient. Instead of feeling frustrated and angry and trying to coerce the patient into submission to the demands, the powerful nurse holds a unit conference to get input from other nurses and to plan care. Through this dialogue, the nurse receives good ideas and all staff members are consistent in their approach with the patient. Manipulative behaviors decrease and the nurse is able to give more effective patient care.

Boyle states, "We accept the idea that power shifts and expands, rather than existing as a limited force. People may then have a great deal of power in some situations and little in others, depending on the goals to be met. Their general power ceases to be of major importance, and their specific power to contribute to meeting our mutual goals becomes the focus. This is a problem-solving approach to the use of power, which is consistent with our use of the professional nursing process. It will enable us to see gaps in power, to recognize those areas in which we need more authority or influence" (p 166).[20]

Cavanaugh's Power Orientations

Heineken used Cavanaugh's Power Orientations when she and Wozniak studied three different levels of nurse managers in order to identify how nurses understand power.[21,22] The three levels of managers included the executive force (*e.g.*, directors, associate directors, and assistant directors of nursing), middle-management (*e.g.*, nursing supervisors), and first-level personnel (*e.g.*, head nurses and charge nurses). The six power orientations as described by Cavanaugh include power as control and autonomy, political, charisma, instinctive drive, resource dependency, and good.[22]

POWER AS CONTROL AND AUTONOMY

Powerholders in this orientation must maintain their independence, autonomy, and control over individuals in the setting through the use of such means as reward and punishment.

POWER AS POLITICAL

In accepting this power orientation, knowing and performing in the system is essential to obtaining and holding power. The basis for this power involves knowing the rules of power and who the players are, both critical requirements in order to "work the system."

POWER AS CHARISMA

In this power orientation a unique social relationship involving a type of drawing power emerges between a person and others. This special magnetism allows the individual to have considerable influence over others.

POWER AS INSTINCTIVE DRIVE

In this type of power orientation the person feels that the wish for power is manifested from within, as an inherent instinct.

POWER AS RESOURCE DEPENDENCY

Resources such as knowledge and information are critical to power in this orientation. This type of power is the result of gaining, maintaining, and carefully allotting resources.

POWER AS GOOD

An individual with this power inherently feels that such power is wanted and admirable.

Heineken reported the outcome of the study by Wozniak and Heineken, "Results showed greatest discrepancy on two power beliefs: (1) power is equated with political abilities and (2) power is associated with the need to maintain control and autonomy. In both instances, nurse executives scored significantly higher than first-level nurse managers. While statistically significant differences did not emerge in the nurse supervisor group, their scores were more closely aligned with the nurse executives on these two power beliefs than with the first-level nurse managers" (p 38).[21]

Heineken cites several implications concerning the results of the study in regard to both power and politics, and power and control/autonomy.[21] She questions if there is not consensus among first-level and top-level management in nursing, how can strategies be planned and implemented in order to affect change? If the concept of power is defined differently between the levels, a real dichotomy could exist with nurse executives being politically astute and head nurses not being concerned at all. The head nurses and charge nurses have considerable influence on patients, families, staff nurses, and other health-care providers; yet, because they put little emphasis on political awareness, "they may miss unique opportunities to gain broad-based support for their ideas, proposals, and programs" (p 38).[21] Head nurses can act as role models for staff nurses; however, if the head nurses do not display political behavior, there will be few chances for staff nurses to observe it. With so many critical issues facing nursing, eventually with this discontinuity any attempt to resolve them will be difficult.[21] This would be true especially when dealing with issues and problems concerning cost containment and cost-effective nursing practices. All nurses must be politically astute in order to control and influence the decisions made concerning these problems, which are nursing problems requiring nursing solutions.

Laws of Power

In addition to being politically clever, it is critical that all nurses learn the laws of power in order to identify and explain strategies to develop power in nursing. Berle discusses the problems in viewing power, which involve both subjective (a facet of human experience) and objective (an actuality in society) factors.[9] It can be as profoundly personal, like love; or it can be immensely and diffusively inclusive. "In its personal aspect, it is a subject for poets and psychologists. In its general aspects, it is a continuing phenomenon of history, politics, and human organization" (p 21).[9]

Berle contends that power is a universal experience.[9] He has identified five natural laws of power. He believes they are usable wherever power exists: whether in a household, business, or government. These laws of power can also be applied to the nurse powerholder: (1) power invariably fills any vacuum in human organization; (2) power is invariably personal; (3) power is invariably based on a system of ideas of philosophy; (4) power is exercised through and depends on institutions; and, (5) power is invariably confronted with, and acts in the presence of, a field of responsibility (p 37).[9] Let us examine these laws in relation to the revolution in the American health care delivery system since the enactment of the prospective payment policy on October 1, 1983.

POWER INVARIABLY FILLS A VACUUM IN HUMAN ORGANIZATION

There is chaos and disorder facing health care providers in regard to cost containment and prospective reimbursement. A real vacuum exists in the power structure of the health care delivery system. Prior to 1983, when retroactive reimbursement was the mode of payment, hospital administrators continued to increase the number of beds; utilized the clinical laboratories and x-ray departments as large revenue-generating areas through the encouraged practice of defensive medicine; and offered services that were diversified and duplicative. With prospective payment (a predetermined amount/case) the "tables are turned," and hospital administrators can no longer use the strategies that were effective with retroactive reimbursement: Chaos exists. Instead of keeping patients in the hospital for as long as possible, the policy is now to get them out as quickly as possible or lose money. The key word in the hospitals is *product management*. The product (*i.e.*, the patient) must be managed in an effective (quality) and efficient (timely) way so that the hospital does not lose money. Hospital boards and administrators are turning to various groups for advice: experts from the business world, physicians, nurses, and others. Chaos exists and there is a real fear of hospitals being closed.

At any class of society, the primary need is for order, not chaos. Peace is a social requisite. Individuals will go to great lengths to have order in their lives both at home and at work. The situation is especially true in hospitals where a power vacuum exists—the question is, who will fill it?

Instinct for power resides, to some extent, in everyone. Although no one ever totally lacks it, power is much stronger in some individuals than in others. When a power vacuum occurs people will move quickly to fill the gap. In engaging in such an action they may meet other individuals who are trying to seize the power. They must defeat the competitor or win them over on their side.

When a vacuum happens within a power structure, power is moved quickly to the next institutional echelon. In the smallest unit, the family, if something happens to the head of the household, another strong family member will take over the leadership functions. The victor of the move in any situation where there is a power vacuum becomes the powerholder.

A combination of three elements creates the powerholders: (1) assertive individuals; (2) an idea that counts; and (3) a group capable of organization. Whenever a vacuum occurs in human organization, it is the brilliance of power to find and fill it.

Nurses hold a pivotal role in patient care delivery within the hospital. They have an idea that not only counts but is popular —to give quality care in the most efficient and effective way. Through cost-effective practices (*i.e.*, goal setting to motivate the patient to early discharge, effective use of supplies, and optimal scheduling) nurses can seize the power. Assertive nurses can express this idea and act as a catalyst to hospital administrators, physicians, and others in their sphere of influence.

Nurses, however, should be guided by our history when asserting their power. Krause[23] notes that nurses have tried in six major ways to fill a power vacuum in health care delivery: (1) the education of nurses moved into the mainstream of higher education in the effort to acquire autonomy; however, nurses still cannot control their practice as physicians in medical school do. Although there are several independent functions in the Nurse Practice Acts, all of the practice involving dependent functions and care in general is under the supervision of the physician. (2) Although it has been approximately 50 years since other members of the nursing team; that is, LPN, nursing assistants, and others emerged on the hospital scene to assist the RNs with their patient care, nurses did not move up in the organizational structure even though some personnel were below them. (3) Nurses moved into positions of management but hospital administrators and physicians had the supreme authority. The management positions were so appealing that non-nurse managers interceded and claimed vast managerial skill. (4) Through the role of a visiting nurse, nurses desired to serve the community; however, hospitals have moved in and bought most of the nurses and their services. (5) Nurses responded to technology and made ICUs and CCUs a prosperous entity; however, hospitals own the technology and physicians control the hospitals. (6) Nurses have worked for power through unionization. The dilemma is that hospitals buy off the nurses with little salary and benefit gains rather than lose any control over patient care. Also, labor unions are moving into the health care arena and offering their services, and to the average staff nurse their price looks good (pp 52–56).[23]

Krause feels that despite failures in the past, nurses can obtain power.[23] In these days of cost containment, the time is ripe for nurses to find power, because of their ideas and their ability to organize, and because nurses are respected in the community.

Sanford assertively states:

> As we move forward, however, to fill the power vacuum in health care, whether it be by an idea about prevention, care of the aged, or something else, we must anticipate that when we make it attractive, others will attempt to wipe us out. We must anticipate that and be prepared to hold our own.
> What if we replaced our "Year of the Nurse" billboards and signs with other signs reading, "Nine out of every ten patients in convalescent hospitals suffer from either bedsores, constipation, depression, incontinence, or perineal rash." It doesn't have to be that way. Ask a registered nurse how these problems can be eliminated through better health care planning . . . Then if need be, the next sign might read, "Guess who doesn't want to eliminate bedsores, constipation, depression, incontinence, and perineal rash?" We're getting lots of pressure from the nursing home industry, physicians, the drug industry, the hospital supplies industry, the paper supplies industry . . . Help us prevent illness! Call 555-2370 (p 18).[24]

Sanford questions whether nurses wouldn't be afraid to confront that much power and money.[24]

Two thirds of the 1.9 million nurses in the United States work in hospitals. Among them there is a cadre of assertive nurses with ideas that matter, who have the ability to organize the health care delivery team in order to fill the power vacuum.

POWER IS INVARIABLY PERSONAL

Power is an inherent quality of man. In the abstract power does not exist. Only when a woman or man instinctively takes and uses it does it become fact. Power does not exist without a powerholder: It is an attitude. Power, however one obtains it, can be used only by the decision and act of a person. Without organization, no elite group, no minority group, no class of people can attain power or use it: In all cases a person is behind that organization. Power is invariably personal.

The right to power occurs through an election or appointment, by an institution, or when a person brings power into being by forming an institution and therefore becomes its leader.

In the mind or hands of a person, the motive toward power is not intrinsically limited. The ability to have others do as you wish has only two limitations: (1) extraneous fact (everything else that's happening in the world) and (2) intellectual or conscience restraint (resolving what you will not or cannot do). The nurse's response as a powerholder will invariably be personal.

Nurses have served society well for years and thus people for the most part trust nurses. They realize that nurses, without a vested interest, have both cared for and about patients. Because of this tradition, the public would probably support nurses as powerholders. The real question is whether or not nurses, knowing that power is invariably personal, will support each other in obtaining power. Norris states, "while pettiness, put-downs, backbiting and sabbotage among nurses are usually blamed on the nature of the interaction among women when they are thrown together, I personally believe that women are as loving and know as much about loving as men — if not more. I believe that their rage, destructiveness, jealousy and intolerance of others' success arises out of centuries of subjugation of women and more than a century of put-downs as nurses . . . We need to restructure our behavior, hard though that is, so that we encourage, foster, indeed demand the movement of our nurse colleagues into status positions, power positions, prestige positions — where they are closer and closer to where the power is and where the real decisions are made."[25]

Nurses can no longer afford not to support and encourage one another when one of them reaches for power. Through role modeling and mentoring head nurses can influence staff nurses in a significant way and encourage each of them to become powerholders in the delivery of cost-effective nursing care. Power is invariably personal.

POWER IS INVARIABLY BASED ON A SYSTEM OF IDEAS OR PHILOSOPHY

Two aspects of power are indivisible. The first is an idea system, a philosophy. The second is an institutional structure capable of transferring the will of the powerholder. Power cannot be produced or disbursed without an institution. The idea must act like a magnet, drawing in followers and obtaining their loyalty, and must generate their time, energy, and money.

Nurses have to focus on the relationship between their practice and the hospital. They need to question the values of the hospital. No values should be more important than quality service. The nurses' idea, or philosophy, centers on the value of caring, which means that the client deserves the best services and that nurses are the best people to develop and manage these services.

Corporate management must be a support system for each head nurse; a channel to communicate experiences, to share ideas, to solve problems, and to anticipate potential outcomes. Nurses, in turn, must become cost-effective managers. Although it may seem like an essential, nurses must believe that nursing is necessary for individuals. They must both monitor productivity and defend the budget. Money and power are closely related and nurses must know where these are to be found, if they are to enter the power arena of health care. A nurse who thinks logically would anticipate that money, time, and energy would be devoted to discovering what quality cost-effective care is. High quality services at reasonable costs is a thought worth great consideration. Will nurses support each other in obtaining power?

POWER IS EXERCISED THROUGH AND DEPENDS ON INSTITUTIONS

In order to exercise power beyond one's personal space, the powerholder must either work through an existing institution or build a new one. An institution does not back a powerholder unless it gets something in return such as considerable time and loving care. The care and feeding of the institution is a major concern of any powerholder.

The person who is the powerholder must remind the institution at all times that she meets a need that no one could fill as well. The delegation of power is also important if the powerholder wants to expand her power.

Sanford is clear in her advice, "Whether we like to face it or not, the nurse must know who to talk to, how to talk to them, and who to call upon to speak for them at the appropriate time. If power is invariably personal, and if power is through and depends on institutions, then we must teach nurses how to mobilize the institutions" (p 22).[24]

Part of the knowledge base nurses need to acquire in order to accomplish this mobilization of institutions includes economics (including health economics), power, and politics, and learning experiences with other health professionals. This continues to be a problem and a responsibility for academia. In the meantime, nurses who do not have these skills must continue their education in order to acquire this knowledge.

The nurse must learn the rules of power in order to be a powerholder, to "play the game," or to win. Historically, women have been defended by society from the harsh truth of the rules of power. Sanford notes, "Physicians, hospital administrators, and college presidents have been all too willing to protect nurses from the harsh realities of the rules of power" (p 23).[24]

For the most part corporate nurse managers know about the rules of power, but what about middle management, head nurses, and staff nurses? How many hospital board of directors have nurses as members? They usually have several physicians serving on the board. This is where the *real* rules of power in any hospital are made.

Nurses are a group that both wants and needs greater participation in formulating the rules of power, so they know what they are, are able to modify them, and win with the rules.

One of the important rules of power in hospitals relates to competition. The competition is fierce between and among hospitals whether they are public, private, nonprofit, or profit making. Marketing strategies and public relations to enhance the image of the hospital are receiving a great deal of attention from hospital administrators and members of the board.

The nursing department has an excellent opportunity to become the competitive edge for a hospital's public relations on a 24-hour basis. This represents a vital link between quality and cost because nurses are in contact with patients 7 days/week, 24 hours/day. Staff nurses can no longer afford to be all things to all people at all times. It is much preferred to have excellence and credibility in select areas rather than to plan and offer several new services. Nurses must have visibility in the community through a market plan that they have developed. Patients will be drawn by quality care as competition increases. Nurses will be intimately involved in developing the rules of power. The value of patient contact, the quality of service, and patient satisfaction are critical elements to such a marketing approach. This opportunity to demonstrate the real value of the professional nurse represents real power for nurses.

POWER IS INVARIABLY CONFRONTED WITH AND ACTS IN THE PRESENCE OF A FIELD OF RESPONSIBILITY

The nurse who is the powerholder must enter the field of responsibility and try to keep power by convincing, deliberating, illustrating, gratifying, or forcing others. This power is personal. The good and bad responses of the individuals in the field of responsibility have a mighty affect on the power holder.

Tension grows when any important group is not part of a communication system. A recognition of the field of responsibility and of the structuring of a communication system within that field, with the powerholder, is what develops a democratic power base. When tension does exist, the powerholder must appear cool, calm, collected, in control, and capable at all times.

Of many factors involved in the field of responsibility, one group, the intellectuals, are especially interesting. Intellectuals usually have an academic background or its equivalent. Because of their knowledge a number of individuals will accept the intellectuals' views.[10]

Nurses who are powerholders in the hospital setting must network with their colleagues in academia. This dialogue will enhance the powerholder's resources. A chasm often exists between nursing practice and nursing education, which is counterproductive to nurses obtaining power. The committee structure in nursing service governance must provide for representation of educators so that through collaboration and unity nursing's field of responsibility will be strengthened.

DEVELOPING PROFESSIONAL AND PERSONAL POWER THROUGH SELF-AWARENESS AND SELF-ESTEEM

It is important that nurses have a positive self-concept and high self-esteem if they expect to be powerholders in meeting the goals of the health care delivery system in a cost-effective way. Nurses can develop both professional and personal power through self-awareness and self-esteem.

Gorton asks several questions in regard to how nurses feel about themselves and their profession.[26] The essence of the questions centers first on the pride that a nurse feels after selecting the nursing profession as a career, and second, on the extent that practicing RNs feel appreciated, frustrated, useless, and powerless. The primary reason for this major change in feelings is influenced by how nurses value themselves; how self-aware they are; and how much self-esteem they have.

Self-awareness is the responsibility of knowing and using what one is.[27] Self-awareness involves how individuals perceive themselves or how they think they relate to others. Nurses need to care for and about themselves before they care for and about others. They are practicing self-awareness when they observe their own feelings and thoughts.

Gorton describes three basic kinds of awareness from a pyramidal model that Stevens developed and places them in a nursing context (Fig. 3-3).[26]

1. *"Awareness of the outside world* is what one sees, hears, smells, tastes, or touches" (p 92).[26] A nurse sees a patient's messy bed, smells the odor of a wound infection, hears the crying of a newborn baby, tastes a salt-free diet, and touches a fevered forehead.

2. *"Awareness of the inside world* means listening to what one's

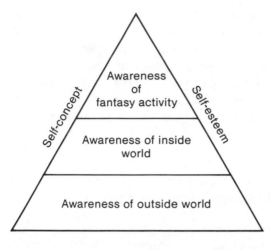

FIGURE 3-3. *Three levels of awareness. (Reproduced with permission from Gorton J: Developing personal power through self-awareness and self-esteem. In Claus K, Bailey J [eds]: Power and Influence in Health Care, p 92. St. Louis, CV Mosby, 1977)*

body is saying — aching, itching, tense, relaxed or hungry" (p 92).[26] A nurse can experience the personal manifestations of euphoria, distress, and emotions.

3. *"Awareness of fantasy activity* occurs when a person knows he is explaining, imagining, interpreting, guessing, thinking, comparing, planning, reminiscing, and anticipating. In formulating future plans or expressing wishes for certain patients (that Mr. G could get out of bed on his own), nurses are using fantasy activity" (p 92).[26]

It is important that nurses develop this third level of awareness and focus their attention on patient care needs, instead of responding only to the outside world of hospital technology or the inside world of their own physical distress.[26]

The strength of one's self-concept relies on the best development of one's own awareness. Self-concept involves the individual's self-image, whereas self-esteem implies how one *feels* about oneself. Self-esteem is of a transitory nature where one may feel good in a particular situation and depressed in another, competent sometimes and incompetent at other times. In order for nurses to feel powerful it is important that they are conscious of the relationship between these messages and aptitudes; otherwise, their self-concept is formed not by their own self-awareness, but by tension exerted on them from the outside.[26]

Gorton identifies three keys for building positive self-concept and high self-esteem.[26]

Key 1. Nurses can Praise Themselves

(a) Self-praise needs practice

Increase self-praise activity in regard to your competent patient care; also, with family and friends.

(b) In absence of objective criteria

Develop an openness for expressing self-praise and satisfaction not objective criteria of self-evaluation; that is, "I feel good about what I did."

(c) Praise selves in both task and environmental situations roles.

Task situation — nurse did a good job. Environmental situation — involved in cost-effective nursing practices

(d) Praise work first then personal qualities.

When trying to convince another person it is easier to accept dispute over one's performance versus one's self-image; in other words, start with, "I changed that dressing well," then move to, "I have a special empathy and patience for patients in pain."

(e) Be specific concerning negative examples.

Instead of constantly criticizing your work in general, which leads to a worthless feeling, be specific about a job that did not meet your expectations and how you will improve the situation.

(f) Don't expect dramatic and immediate changes in yourself.

If you regard yourself as a failure any difficulty encountered then confirms your self-concept. Think and act positively. Difficulties are only "stepping stones" to success as a powerholder.

Key 2. Nurses Can Set Realistic Goals

(a) Personal goals	It is important that you set your own goals; that you are committed to them; and that you evaluate how well you achieved them.
(b) Goals based on performance	Set each goal a little higher each day, and you will be more motivated to reach it.
(c) Attainable goals	This involves short- and long-term goals. Short-term goals should be attainable. Long-term goals should be attainable and realistic.

Key 3. Nurses Can Evaluate Realistically

Nurses must evaluate themselves correctly and realistically in order to improve their self-concept and self-esteem. Evaluations should be based on progress over past performance, not unrealistic goals. Everyone makes mistakes; no one is perfect all the time. Nurses with high self-esteem recognize their deficiencies but do not dwell on them; rather, they work steadily to improve them.

It is important that nurses have a positive self-concept and high self-esteem if they expect to be powerholders. Gorton's three keys and the exercises that follow are useful tools for nurses in realizing achievement in this area.[26]

Gorton's Exercises*

1. *Awareness.* Dosage: three times a day for 2 minutes each session. Take the time to pay attention to your awareness now and two other times today at work and at home. Be an observer of your awareness and notice where it goes. Say to yourself, "Now I'm aware of . . ." and finish this sentence with what you are aware of at the moment and then notice whether this is something outside, something inside, or a fantasy. Where does your awareness go? Are you mostly

*Reproduced with permission from Gorton J: Developing personal power through self-awareness and self-esteem. In Claus K, Bailey J (eds): Power and Influence in Health Care. St. Louis, CV Mosby, 1977

aware of things outside your body or sensations inside your skin?

Now I am aware of . . .

Now I am aware of . . .

Now I am aware of . . .

Now direct your attention to whichever area you are least aware of, inside or outside, and become aware of this. To what extent are you occupied with fantasies, thoughts, and images? Notice that while you are occupied with a thought or an image, your awareness of inside and outside reality decreases or disappears. Are you occupied with fantasies, thoughts, and images more at work or more at home?

2. *Awareness at home.* Dosage: 3 minutes when you first come home. Now sit down and close your eyes and experience what it was like to be there at work. Ask yourself the following questions:

What was it like to be there?

How do you feel there?

How do people appear there?

Who do you feel uncomfortable with there?

What noises do you hear there?

What colors do you see there?

Are you able to leave what was there at work and be in the here of home?

3. *Awareness at work.* Dosage: 3 minutes when you first arrive at work. Look around you and get in touch with your surroundings. What do you experience here?

What is it like to be here?

How do you feel here?

How do the people appear here?

With whom do you feel uncomfortable?

With whom do you feel comfortable?

What noises do you hear?

What colors do you see?

Practicing Self-Praise

Dosage: 15 minutes at coffee break.

1. While you're sipping your coffee, write down (as quickly as

possible) all the things you feel "good" about having done today.

> I feel good about . . .
>
> I feel good about . . .
>
> I feel good about . . .

2. Next, write down how you contributed to making your ward run efficiently.

> I helped things run smoothly by . . .
>
> I helped things run smoothly by . . .
>
> I helped things run smoothly by . . .

3. Now write down what you like about yourself at work.

> I like the way I . . .
>
> I like the way I . . .
>
> I like the way I . . .

See if what you feel good about in no. 1 is also the role you like and use to make your unit run smoothly. Was it easier to praise your work than yourself?

Setting Realistic Goals

Dosage: every day.

1. Every day before you start work write down one goal you have for that day that is unique to you.

> My personal goal for today is to . . .

2. Now, state your goal so that it is unique to you and is in relation to your past performance.

> The weaknesses I wish to build on today are . . .
>
> The strengths I wish to develop are . . .

3. Next, state your goal so that it is personal, accounts for your past abilities, and sets an obtainable standard for today.

> Yesterday's performance tells me that my new goal for today is to improve . . .

Evaluating Your Performance

1. Dosage: every day after work. Examine how you are working now compared to one of your past performances.

> Compared to how I worked when I first started this job, I now . . .
>
> At the beginning of a shift I . . . compared to my performance of . . . at the end of a shift.

Two weeks ago I . . . and now I . . .

2. Dosage: every time you face a unique task. Evaluate how well you do separate tasks.

I can administer medications . . .

My nursing care consists of . . .

When communicating with physicians . . .

3. Dosage: every time you have a new task or try to change your work habits. Evaluate your work in terms of how you are improving.

I am improving my . . .

The first step I've taken toward success in . . .

Today I successfully moved toward . . .

Implications and Application for Nurses: Guideline for Action

The concept of power is nebulous: it is hard to define. However, nurses can take steps become more powerful. The following steps represent a guideline for action.

Step 1. Develop an awareness and understanding of power. Learn more about power by reading and by observing the actions of individuals you consider powerful, both personally and professionally. Keep your "power antenna" receptive.

Step 2. Use Gorton's tools and exercises for self-awareness and self-esteem.[26] Follow the instructions for these tools and exercises so that you become more self-confident and unafraid of power. Feel good and think positively about being an RN in these days of cost containment.

Step 3. Collaborate with your colleagues on cost-effective nursing practices. Nurses make an impact on patients through expert power; however, they are deficient on cost issues and how they impact on hospital finances. Examine what you know and do in this regard and discuss it with your colleagues so that you can develop expert power in areas related to costs.

Step 4. Identify the nurses with the most influence (power) on your unit. Be aware of the use, abuse, and misuse of supplies and equipment. Form a small group of nurses who want to reduce the costs in this area. Act as a catalyst and influence other nurses to follow your lead. Monitor the results over 3 months. Send the results of your efforts (savings to hospital and patient) to top level administration.

Step 5. Review the types of power: Reward, coercive, legitimate, referent, and expert. Keep a daily journal indicating what type, how often, in what situation, and what results you got in terms of influencing another individual's behavior when using the various types of power. Determine which type is most effective for you, especially in cost-effective nursing practices. Look closely at three areas of your influence: goal setting for the patient, effective use of supplies by your colleagues, and optimal scheduling of patients involving health professionals from other departments.

Step 6. Review the by-laws of the nursing department and the hospital. Check the membership of the committees and which level of nurses are involved. This not only includes the quality control committee, but also the finance committee and the board of directors. Work through nursing service to ensure there is two-way communication, input, and influence. *You* can thus help to make the rules of the game and gain power.

Questions for Reflection and Discussion

1. How important do you think power is for a nurse to have in giving cost-effective patient care?

2. Do you believe that a few nurses, in a short time, could make a dramatic difference in the way that care is given in your hospital? Who should the nurses be in terms of level or type?

3. How powerful do you feel the nurses on your unit are and how could you enhance their power?

4. What are the strengths and areas of concern of the Blaney/Hobson integrated model of power within the context of cost-effective nursing practice?

5. Which type of power do you prefer to use in dealing with people?

6. Do you believe that nurses do not have more expert power than physicians in the delivery of patient care?

7. Are more of the nurses you work with blue-collar or white-collar workers? How does it affect patient care on your unit?

8. How often do nurses in your unit collaborate in discussions of knowledge, skills, and attitudes concerning the scope of their practice? Do you feel this collective action would increase both your power and the power of nursing?

9. Is it important that head nurses and staff nurses be as politically astute as the top-level nursing management?

10. Do you believe it is important to know the rules of power in your hospital? Do you think nurses are powerful enough on your unit to "fill the vacuum" in your hospital organization if one exists in regard to cost containment?

11. How well is your awareness of fantasy activity developed and how could you improve yourself in this area?

12. How useful did you find the Gorton exercises on self-awareness? Have they increased your self-awareness, self-concept, self-esteem, or self-confidence?

REFERENCES

1. Kalisch PA, Kalish BJ: The Advance of American Nursing. Boston, Little, Brown, 1978
2. Ashley JA: This I believe about power in nursing. Nurs Dimensions 7:28–32, 1979
3. Lasswell HD: Power and Personality, pp 39–44. New York, WW Norton, 1948
4. Mills CW: The Power Elite. New York, Oxford University Press, 1956
5. Grissum M, Spengler C: Women, Power and Health Care. Boston, Little, Brown, 1976
6. Hawley AH: Community power and urban renewal success. Am J Sociol 2:422–431, 1968
7. Kalisch BJ, Kalisch PA: Politics of Nursing. Philadelphia, JB Lippincott, 1982
8. Mechanic D: Sources of power of lower participants in complex organization. Admin Sci Q 7:349–362, 1962
9. Berle A: Power. New York, Harcourt, Brace, & World, 1969
10. Craig JH, Craig M: Synergic Power: Beyond Domination and Permissiveness. Berkley, CA, Proactive Press, 1974
11. Claus K, Bailey I: Power and Influence in Health Care. St. Louis, CV Mosby, 1977
12. Harsanyi J: Measurement of social power, opportunity costs, and the theory of two-person bargaining games. Behav Sci 7:67–80, 1962
13. French J, Raven B: Basis of social power. In Cartwright D, Zander A (eds): Group Dynamics Research and Theory, 3rd ed, pp 259–269. New York, Harper & Row, 1968
14. Wolf MS: Power in nursing: Group theories perspective. In Wiec-

zorek R (ed): Power, Politics, and Policy in Nursing. New York, Springer, 1985
15. Kirkpatrick JJ: Political Woman. New York, Basic Books, 1974
16. Petro CS, Putnam BA: Sex-role stereotypes: Issues of attitudinal changes. Sex Roles: A Journal of Research 5:29–39, 1979
17. McClure M: Managing the professional nurse. Paper presented at the Journal of Nursing Administration (JONA) Conference, New York, 1980
18. Smith ED: Career versus job orientation: A power dilemma in nursing and feminism. In Wieczorek R (ed): Power, Politics, and Policy in Nursing. New York, Springer, 1985
19. Garant C: Power, leadership, and nursing. Nurs Forum 20:183–199, 1981
20. Boyle K: Power in nursing: A collaborative approach. Nurs Outlook 32:164–167, 1984
21. Heineken J: Power, conflicting views. J Nurs Admin 15:36–39, 1985
22. Cavanaugh MA: A formulative investigation of power orientation and preliminary validation of relationships between power orientations and communication. Doctoral dissertation. University of Denver, 1979
23. Krause EA: Power and Illness. New York, Elsevier North–Holland, 1977
24. Sanford N: Identification and explanation of strategies to develop power for nursing. In Power, Nursing's Challenge for Change. American Nurses' Association, 1979
25. Norris CM: The survival of nursing 1975 and beyond. Paper presented to the California Nurses' Association, Region 10, Fort Ord, CA, May 17, 1975
26. Gorton J: Developing personal power through self-awareness and self-esteem. In Claus K, Bailey J (eds): Power and Influence in Health Care. St. Louis, CV Mosby, 1977
27. Perls F, Hefferline RF, Goodman P: Gestalt Therapy: Excitement and Growth in the Human Personality. New York, Julian Press, 1951

4

Measurement and Improvement of Nursing Attitudes Toward Cost-Effectiveness

THE ISSUE of cost-effectiveness in health care has received a great deal of attention in recent years. The pressure for increased efficiency has been felt throughout the health care delivery system, including the important area of nursing care.

Given the prominence and significance of cost-effectiveness, nurses have developed feelings or attitudes regarding this issue. The development of these attitudes is influenced by incidents and cases reported in the media, highlighting failures of the system. Anyone in the nursing profession is aware of examples in which the overzealous pursuit of cost-effectiveness objectives has resulted in poor quality patient care, and in some serious cases, even complicating conditions and death. These abuses, combined with reports of patients being denied medical care because of an inability to pay, create a negative image of cost-effectiveness efforts.

In addition, within the nursing profession, cost-effectiveness is often associated with several other negative factors, including staffing reductions, salary or pay cuts, working longer and harder, and reductions in support resources. Consequently, it is not surprising to find that many nurses have less-than-positive attitudes toward the issue of cost-effectiveness.

Why is a positive attitude toward cost-effectiveness important in nursing? As indicated in Chapter 1, cost issues for hospitals have rapidly become survival issues. Given that the continued importance of providing patient care is the mission of most hospitals and the nurse's focal role in this process, nursing behaviors and practice must become more cost-effective. Improvements in nursing are essential for the financial health and continued operation of many hospitals.

Although a person's behavior with respect to a particular issue is influenced by many interrelated factors, a major determinant is the individual's attitude toward the issue involved. A significant body of behavioral science research has confirmed this attitude/behavior link.

For nurses, this means that cost-effective behaviors are influenced significantly by their attitudes toward the issue in general. If nurses' attitudes are negative, the development of appropriate behaviors will be difficult. On the other hand, positive attitudes toward cost-effectiveness will facilitate the process of acquiring, implementing, and using more cost-effective behaviors.

Ideally, then, cost-effectiveness programs should be preceded by an assessment of the prevailing attitude toward this issue. If attitudes are negative, attempts to improve them should precede the actual program. A failure to reverse negative attitudes will significantly increase the probability of program failure. Where prevailing attitudes are positive, cost-effectiveness programs can be initiated immediately without first addressing the attitudinal component.

Unfortunately, until recently, the importance of attitudes toward cost-effectiveness has been overlooked in the nursing literature and no attitude assessment instruments have been available. The need for theory, research, and practical applications in this area is critical. The material contained in this chapter will hopefully stimulate and facilitate these efforts.

The purpose of this chapter is fourfold: (1) to familiarize nurses with the concept of attitude and relate it to the issue of cost-effectiveness, (2) to present the widely supported Fishbein and Ajzen model of the attitude process, (3) to introduce the newly developed and successfully tested Blaney/Hobson Nursing Attitude Scale as a reliable and valid tool to measure attitudes toward cost-effectiveness might plan or intend to carry out her tude change strategies and offer practical suggestions for nursing.

ATTITUDE DEFINITION AND CONCEPTUAL MODEL

The concept of *attitude* has been one of the most important and widely researched topics in the field of social psychology.[1] Although the term has been variously defined over the years,[2] there is now general agreement that attitude refers to a predisposition to respond in a favorable or unfavorable manner towards an object, person, or concept; in other words, an attitude reflects our feelings about a particular topic.

Basic Assumptions

Several important assumptions underly this definition of attitude. First, an attitude represents a hypothetical construct that cannot be observed directly, but is something that exists inside people. Although we can evaluate the behavioral consequences of an attitude, we cannot see the attitude itself.

Second, an attitude is a unidimensional variable. This means that attitudes are measured on a single continuum of favorability—from very unfavorable to very favorable. Attitudes reflect the way we feel about a particular topic and represent our emotional response on a scale from bad to good.

Third, although attitudes cannot be observed directly, they can be measured accurately. Several techniques have been developed to allow for the accurate assessment of a person's attitude. These techniques generally involve some form of written questionnaire. (A scale developed to specifically measure nursing attitude towards cost-effectiveness is presented later in this chapter.)

Fourth, attitudes are learned as a result of the socialization process. Major influences on the development of one's attitudes include the overall culture or society, the family, co-workers, friends, major groups to which one belongs, and prior work experiences. In addition, formal education and the media impact on attitude development. The essential point is that attitudes represent the result of a basic learning process.

A fifth assumption is that attitudes are related to subsequent behavior. Although this relationship is far from perfect, there is considerable evidence that attitudes are a major determinant of a person's behavior.[3-6] One's attitude toward a person, object, or concept is a reasonably good indicator of how an individual will actually behave.

Fishbein and Ajzen Attitude Model

Probably the most widely accepted, well-formulated, and research-supported attitude model is the model developed by Fishbein and Ajzen.[7] This model, shown in Figure 4-1, conceptualizes the attitude process as consisting of four basic components: beliefs, attitudes, behavioral intentions, and actual behaviors, arranged in a causal sequence.

Beliefs are defined as statements held to be true and factual concerning the characteristics associated with a particular object, person, or concept. For instance, the following is a belief concerning cost-effectiveness in nursing: cost-effectiveness leads to poor quality patient care. According to Fishbein and Ajzen, such evaluative beliefs lead directly to the development of a person's attitude toward that topic. Beliefs therefore form the

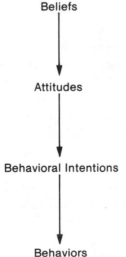

FIGURE 4-1. *Fishbein and Ajzen attitude model. (Adapted from Fishbein M, Ajzen I: Belief, Attitude, Intention, and Behavior: An Introduction to Theory and Research. Reading, MA, Addison–Wesley, 1975)*

underlying basis of attitudes. As beliefs about an object are formed, an attitude toward the object begins to evolve slowly.

In the Fishbein and Ajzen model, the term *attitude* refers specifically to a learned predisposition to respond in a consistently favorable or unfavorable manner toward a particular object. This is essentially the same definition given for attitude and is generally accepted. Again, an attitude refers to how a person feels about a particular topic on a continuum of favorability. Within this model, one's attitude depends on one's set of beliefs held concerning the attitude – object. For example, a nurse's attitude toward cost-effectiveness is a function of her beliefs about this issue and its consequences for nursing.

As the Fishbein and Ajzen model indicates, attitudes do not lead directly to actual behaviors, but instead lead first to the development of behavioral intentions. These intentions consist of a person's planned or intended response to a particular object (*i.e.*, how a person intends to behave).

Behavioral intentions are postulated to be a direct result of one's attitude. For instance, a nurse with a favorable attitude toward cost-effectiveness might plan or intend to carry out her duties in a cost-effective manner. The model illustrates that such behavioral intentions are the direct cause of a person's actual behavior. Thus, although attitudes are not related directly in a causal sense to actual behaviors, there is a strong link between attitudes and behavior through the development and functioning of one's behavioral intentions.

As mentioned earlier, the Fishbein and Ajzen attitude model has received broad research support and widespread acceptability.[7] Several important implications for nursing can be derived from this model and the preceding general discussion of attitudes.

Nursing Implications

Although the concept of attitude has many potentially significant implications for nurses interested in improving cost-effectiveness, the following are especially important:

1. Virtually all nurses have by now developed an attitude towards the issue of cost-effectiveness.

2. These nursing attitudes are based on beliefs about cost-effectiveness and its consequences.

3. When cost-effectiveness is believed to lead to several negative outcomes (*i.e.*, lower quality patient care, more work, fewer resources), correspondingly negative attitudes will develop.

4. Given the causal relationship from attitude → behavioral intention → behavior, a negative nursing attitude toward cost-effectiveness can present a significant obstacle to the success of efforts to improve behaviors in this area.

5. Recognizing the importance of nursing attitudes, comprehensive efforts to improve cost-effective behaviors should first begin with an assessment of the prevailing attitudes. When nursing attitudes are positive, behavioral improvement strategies can be initiated with a strong expectation of success. Negative attitudes, however, will make it difficult to improve nursing behaviors. In such situations, a concerted effort to substantially improve nursing attitudes is needed first.

6. In order to be able to accurately assess nursing attitudes toward cost-effectiveness, it is necessary to develop a reliable and valid measurement tool.

These implications are significant particularly for nurses interested in improving the cost-effectiveness of nursing practice. Success in this endeavor hinges on the development of positive attitudes. In the next section, a new measurement tool to measure nursing attitudes toward cost-effectiveness is presented, followed by a discussion of how to improve attitudes when they are less than positive.

BLANEY/HOBSON NURSING ATTITUDE SCALE

Efforts to improve the cost-effectiveness of nursing behaviors should be preceded by an assessment of nursing attitudes towards this issue. However, until recently, no reliable and valid measurement tool has been available. A research program was initiated in 1984 at Indiana University Northwest to address this need, and to develop and evaluate a tool designed specifically to measure nursing attitude toward cost-effectiveness. This program was part of a larger project sponsored by the University of Maryland, dealing with the measurement of clinical and educational nursing outcomes. The research effort resulted in the construction of the Blaney/Hobson Nursing Attitude Scale.

The 20-item scale is presented in the box, Blaney/Hobson Nursing Attitude Scale. Complete the questionnaire before con-

BLANEY/HOBSON NURSING ATTITUDE SCALE

Directions

Please respond to the following statements dealing with the issue of cost-effectiveness in nursing practices and procedures by indicating the extent to which you disagree or agree with each one. Please *circle* your response.

	Strongly Disagree	Disagree Somewhat	Neither Agree Nor Disagree	Agree Somewhat	Strongly Agree
1. The introduction and use of cost-effective practices and procedures will improve overall nursing effectiveness.	SD	D	N	A	SA
2. The introduction and use of cost-effective nursing practices and procedures will benefit me personally.	SD	D	N	A	SA
3. Operating a nursing unit in order to make a profit is wrong.	SD	D	N	A	SA
4. I look forward to the introduction and use of cost-effective practices and procedures in nursing.	SD	D	N	A	SA
5. The introduction and use of cost-effective nursing practices and procedures will result in a decrease in the quality of patient care.	SD	D	N	A	SA
6. The introduction and use of cost-effective practices and procedures will benefit the nursing profession as a whole.	SD	D	N	A	SA

(Continued)

BLANEY/HOBSON NURSING ATTITUDE SCALE *(Continued)*

Directions

Please respond to the following statements dealing with the issue of cost-effectiveness in nursing practices and procedures by indicating the extent to which you disagree or agree with each one. Please *circle* your response.

	Strongly Disagree	Disagree Somewhat	Neither Agree Nor Disagree	Agree Somewhat	Strongly Agree
7. The thought of introducing "cost-effectiveness" into nursing makes me uneasy.	SD	D	N	A	SA
8. Hospital nursing units should not be concerned with making or losing money.	SD	D	N	A	SA
9. The introduction and use of cost-effective nursing practices and procedures will benefit patients.	SD	D	N	A	SA
10. Nurses should not be obligated to provide patient care in a cost-effective manner.	SD	D	N	A	SA
11. I look forward to learning more about cost-effectiveness in nursing.	SD	D	N	A	SA
12. Cost-effectiveness goes against the basic principles of good nursing.	SD	D	N	A	SA
13. The whole idea of cost-effectiveness in nursing upsets me.	SD	D	N	A	SA
14. Cost-effectiveness is bad for nursing.	SD	D	N	A	SA
15. I feel good when I save the hospital money.	SD	D	N	A	SA

(Continued)

BLANEY/HOBSON NURSING ATTITUDE SCALE *(Continued)*

Directions

Please respond to the following statements dealing with the issue of cost-effectiveness in nursing practices and procedures by indicating the extent to which you disagree or agree with each one. Please *circle* your response.

	Strongly Disagree	Disagree Somewhat	Neither Agree Nor Disagree	Agree Somewhat	Strongly Agree
16. I welcome the new emphasis on cost-effectiveness in nursing.	SD	D	N	A	SA
17. Cost-effectiveness programs only mean more work for nurses.	SD	D	N	A	SA
18. Cost-effectiveness programs are a hassle for nurses.	SD	D	N	A	SA
19. Learning more about cost-effectiveness will help me be a better nurse.	SD	D	N	A	SA
20. I fully agree with the need to improve cost-effectiveness in nursing.	SD	D	N	A	SA

(Copyright, 1985. Reprinted with permission from Blaney DR and Hobson CJ.)

sidering the format, scoring and interpretation, psychometric characteristics, and appropriate use of the tool. Respond to each item by circling your answer, using the 5-point scale from "strongly disagree" to "strongly agree."

Best results for this scale are obtained when people respond to the questions as truthfully and honestly as possible. Answer quickly and do not spend time pondering over each one. Read the question carefully and then answer it in the way you feel about it. Put down your first reaction and then continue to the next question. When you have completed all 20 items, turn to the box, Blaney/Hobson Nursing Attitude Scale Scoring Instructions, for the self-scoring instructions. Follow these instructions closely

---

BLANEY/HOBSON NURSING ATTITUDE SCALE SCORING INSTRUCTIONS

Scoring Instructions

The questionnaire consists of 20 items. Two procedures are used in scoring the results.

For the following ten items, use Scoring Procedure 1 and write the score for each item in the blank preceding that item.

Items	*Scoring Procedure 1*
Item 1	SD = 1
Item 2	D = 2
Item 4	N = 3
Item 6	A = 4
Item 9	SA = 5
Item 11	
Item 15	
Item 16	
Item 19	
Item 20	

For the remaining ten items below, use Scoring Procedure 2 and write the score for each item in the blank preceding that item.

Items	*Scoring Procedure 2*
Item 3	SD = 5
Item 5	D = 4
Item 7	N = 3
Item 8	A = 2
Item 10	SA = 1
Item 12	
Item 13	
Item 14	
Item 17	
Item 18	

When you have written the score for each item in the blank preceding that item, the next step involves adding up these scores for the 20 items in the questionnaire. This will give you your overall score.

On the questionnaire, scores can range from a low of 20 to a high of 100, with an average of 60. The higher your score, the more positive your attitude toward cost-effectiveness in nursing.

A = agree somewhat; D = disagree somewhat; N = neither agree nor disagree; SA = strongly agree; SD = strongly disagree. (Copyright, 1985. Reprinted with permission from Blaney DR and Hobson CJ.)

---

and you will obtain your overall score on the scale. Basic interpretative guidelines are also provided.

Now that you know what your own score is, more detailed information about scale format, scoring and interpretation, psychometric characteristics, and appropriate utilization will be provided.

Scale Format

Many alternative attitude measurement models and formats are available in the literature. In constructing the Blaney/Hobson Nursing Attitude Scale, the popular Likert model of "summated ratings" was chosen for use,[8] due to its straightforward developmental and analytical procedures and strong reliability and validity.

The Likert format involves measuring attitudes by asking people to respond to a series of statements by indicating the extent to which they agree or disagree with each one. The Blaney/Hobson Nursing Attitude Scale consists of 20 such items and uses a response format with 5 categories, ranging from "strongly disagree" to "strongly agree."

Scoring and Interpretation

Within Likert's summated ratings model, a person's response to each individual item is scored. These item scores are then totaled to provide an overall measure of their attitude. For scoring purposes on the Blaney/Hobson Nursing Attitude Scale, a 5-point scheme was used for each item. For example, "strongly disagree" counts for one point, "disagree somewhat" counts for two points, and so on through "strongly agree," which counts for five points.

In order for this scoring procedure to function properly, any negatively worded items must first be "reverse scored." This means that the scoring system is reversed for any negatively worded item. In other words, "strongly disagree" as a response to a negatively worded statement would be scored as a very positive five points.

For example, on the scale, item number 7 states, "the thought of introducing 'cost-effectiveness' into nursing makes me uneasy." This item represents a negatively worded statement — cost-effectiveness leads to a negative outcome, a feeling of uneasiness. A person responding "strongly disagree" to this item is expressing a very positive attitude towards cost-effectiveness, and thus that person's score for that item would be five. Had he responded "disagree somewhat," his score would have been four, and so on through a response of "strongly agree," which would have resulted in a score of one.

A total of ten negatively worded items were included on the Blaney/Hobson Nursing Attitude Scale — items 3, 5, 7, 8, 10, 12, 13, 14, 17, and 18. After reverse scoring these items, a person's total score is obtained by simply adding up the 20 individual item scores.

The maximum possible score is 100, the minimum is 20, and the midpoint is 60. Higher scores indicate a more positive attitude towards cost-effectiveness. Scores below 60 suggest a generally negative attitude, whereas scores above 60 reflect a positive attitude. You can interpret your own personal score in terms of these guidelines.

Psychometric Characteristics

The potential use of any attitude scale must be evaluated in terms of its underlying psychometric characteristics. Psychometrics is a field of study involving the measurement of psychological variables such as traits, mental abilities, attitudes, emotions, and opinions. Theory and research in this field confirm that a useful psychological measurement tool must have two critical psychometric characteristics: reliability and validity.[9]

Reliability refers to the consistency with which a measurement is made. For example, assume that a thermometer is properly used to take a healthy person's temperature under the same conditions two times within a 10-minute span. If the first reading is 99.4 and the second is 97.3, the thermometer is not providing reliable or consistent results; as such, it is useless as a measuring device. Similarly, an attitude scale must provide reliable, consistent measurements or it is also useless.

Rigorous research studies have been conducted with the Blaney/Hobson Nursing Attitude Scale to evaluate its reliability.[10] The results of this continuing research indicate that the scale is a highly reliable measurement tool and well exceeds the minimum standards for acceptable reliability adopted by psychometricians.[9] Thus, one can conclude that the scale is a reliable and consistent measure of nursing attitude towards cost-effectiveness.

Validity is the second essential characteristic that an effective attitude scale must possess. It refers to the extent to which a scale measures what it is designed to measure; that is, does the Blaney/Hobson Nursing Attitude Scale measure nursing attitude toward cost-effectiveness?

Extensive (and continuing) research has been conducted to assess the validity of the scale, and the results have been strongly supportive. Three examples are discussed to illustrate the nature of this research. First, a statistically significant relationship (positive correlation) has been found between attitude scores and measures of cost-effective job performance. Nurses with more positive attitudes generally tend to perform their jobs in a more cost-effective manner.

Second, the presentation of a training program designed to improve nursing attitudes towards cost-effectiveness resulted in a statistically significant improvement in scores on the Blaney/ Hobson Nursing Attitude Scale. A large group of hospital nurses completed the scale both before and after the training program for comparison purposes. The data indicate that the scale is accurately measuring nursing attitudes by virtue of its sensitivity to the content and purpose of the training program.

Finally, the scale has been administered to three distinct subgroups within the nursing profession — staff nurses, head nurses, and nurse administrators. If the scale does accurately measure nursing attitudes toward cost-effectiveness, one would expect to find that the average score is highest in the nurse administrator group, next highest in the head nurse group, and lowest in the staff nurse group. Although there are many plausible rationales for this hypothesis, a major one is that nurses in supervisory and administrative positions must by necessity adopt a more positive attitude towards cost-effectiveness given the requirements of their jobs and their responsibility for cost-related aspects of nursing practice.

The data collected using the Blaney/Hobson Nursing Attitude Scale reveal significant differences in the average attitude levels of the three groups. Attitudes are most positive in the nurse administrator group, least positive among staff nurses, with head nurses in between the two. These results strongly confirm the aforementioned hypothesis.

The combined results of the research on the Blaney/Hobson Nursing Attitude Scale demonstrate that it possesses the required psychometric characteristics of strong reliability and validity. The scale provides a consistent and accurate means of measuring nursing attitudes toward cost-effectiveness.

Scale Utilization

Given the availability of a reliable and valid tool to measure nursing attitudes, several potentially important uses of the scale are possible. First, as part of a comprehensive training approach to improve the cost-effectiveness of nursing practice, the Blaney/Hobson Nursing Attitude Scale can be ideally used to initially assess the attitude level of the target nursing group. Information collected in this manner has important implications for the actual content of the training program. For example, a strong negative attitude would suggest that specific steps to improve nursing attitudes must be developed and implemented in order for subsequent behavioral change strategies to be successful. On the other hand, if attitude scores are uniformly positive, behavioral training efforts could proceed immediately, with a high probability of success.

The link between attitudes and behavior is so strong that poor attitudes will seriously limit, or in some cases, totally negate the impact of behavioral improvement programs. In other words, if nurses exhibit a negative attitude towards cost-effectiveness, direct attempts to improve nursing performance behaviors will likely meet with failure. Consequently, when negative attitudes are present, they must be dealt with explicitly, prior to addressing desired behavioral changes. Research documented methods to improve attitudes are presented in the next section.

While the Blaney/Hobson Nursing Attitude Scale should ideally be used as the first step in a comprehensive program to improve the cost-effectiveness of nursing practice, it can also be used where such programs have already been initiated, yet are not producing the desired outcomes. One likely cause of failure in these instances is the existence of strong negative attitudes. Information relevant to this potential obstacle can be obtained by administering the Blaney/Hobson Nursing Attitude Scale. If scores are low, a major revision in training strategy is required and should involve a concerted effort to first improve attitudes before addressing desired behavioral changes. If scale scores are high, other causes of program failure must be investigated.

Most hospitals have already initiated some type of program designed to improve the cost-effectiveness of nursing practice. These efforts have met with varying degrees of success. Given the close link between attitudes and behaviors, a possible reason contributing to the relative failure of many programs is the presence of strong negative attitudes on the part of the nurses involved. Thus, nursing managers are advised to address this issue specifically by using the Blaney/Hobson Nursing Attitude

Scale and by formulating training strategies based on its results. Periodic administration of the scale would allow nurse managers to monitor prevailing attitudes towards cost-effectiveness and identify potential problems before they become serious.

Finally, a third potential use of the Blaney/Hobson Nursing Attitude Scale is as a screening device in the hiring process. In view of the growing importance of financial considerations in health care, nursing units can no longer afford to hire individuals with poor attitudes toward cost-effectiveness. Thus, given a choice between two equally qualified nurses, differing only in their attitude towards cost issues, most nurse managers would probably choose the one with the more positive attitude.

As revolutionary and radical as this may seem, the "rules of the game" have changed dramatically and permanently. In the modern health care setting, the successful nurse can no longer be oblivious to or antagonistic toward cost issues. The Blaney/Hobson Nursing Attitude Scale can be used as a tool in the hiring process to make decisions about applicants on this dimension of critical and growing importance.

ATTITUDE IMPROVEMENT STRATEGIES

Extensive research has been conducted in social psychology on the various strategies designed to change or improve attitudes.[5,11,12] In this section, several of the more effective approaches are introduced and discussed under three major headings: (1) message characteristics, (2) communicator characteristics, and (3) perceived outcome factors. The most effective attitude change strategies include as many of these approaches as possible.

Message Characteristics

A primary focus of research in attitude change processes has been on the characteristics of the message intended to effect the change. This research has led to the identification of several important factors that enhance the efficacy of an attitude change message. Four of the most significant of these factors are listed in the box, Important Message Characteristics in Attitude Improvement.

First, evidence shows that people in many cases develop atti-

---

IMPORTANT MESSAGE CHARACTERISTICS IN ATTITUDE IMPROVEMENT

1. Factual, complete, relevant, current information
2. Simple, well-organized, straightforward structure
3. Two-sided presentation with both advantages and disadvantages
4. Frequent repetition of the basic message

---

tudes on the basis of incomplete and inaccurate information. This has undoubtedly occurred in the area of cost-effectiveness in nursing. Negative attitudes are often formed on the basis of sketchy information of questionable accuracy and completeness.

Given this fairly common phenomena, it is not surprising then that a powerful way to improve attitudes simply involves the presentation of factual, complete, relevant, and current information regarding the focal issue. In applying this principle to nursing, attitudes can be improved by providing accurate and comprehensive data regarding cost-effectiveness techniques and their use and implementation. Using this approach, ignorance, fear of the unknown, and distorted perceptions as contributing causes to a poor attitude can be minimized.

A second important message characteristic is the complexity and organizational structure of the content. Research has shown that attitude change is more likely to be initiated by simple, straightforward, well-organized messages. People seem to be able to better understand, remember, and respond to such messages. At a basic level, attitude change cannot be expected to result from a message that is too complex or disorganized to understand.

Attempts to improve nursing attitudes would be well advised to follow this simple advice and avoid overly complicated and disjointed messages. For example, a presentation consisting of concepts and terminology in accounting, budgeting, and business cost-control strategies is probably not appropriate for most nurses. Without the necessary background, such a presentation would be difficult to understand. Simplicity is a virtue in attitude change messages. Effective presentations should build on a nurse's knowledge base and introduce cost concepts in the most straightforward manner possible. The information in this chapter represents an attempt to present some of the basic concepts in cost control, without assuming any prior knowledge in this area. It is sufficient to say that advanced, sophisticated, and poorly organized attitude change messages are not effective in improving nursing attitudes.

A third message characteristic that plays a significant role in mediating attitude change concerns the debate over whether both sides of a position should be presented or only the positive side. Should both the potential advantages and disadvantages of cost-effectiveness in nursing be presented, or should the message only address the advantages?

Research findings suggest that greater attitude change occurs when two-sided messages are used, especially when the target group is experienced, interested, and involved with the issue. Presenting both sides of an issue creates an impression of honesty, objectivity, realism, and even-handedness. This results generally in a more favorable response to the underlying message.

The application of this principle is obvious and clear-cut in nursing. Attempts to improve nursing attitude toward cost-effectiveness should definitely include a consideration of both the advantages and disadvantages. Arguing that cost-effectiveness only leads to positive outcomes for nurses will result in poor message acceptance.

Most nurses are familiar with the problems that can be caused by cost-effectiveness efforts and these potential problems, such as lower quality care, reduced staffing, and heavier work loads, should be explicitly acknowledged and dealt with. In this manner, negative feelings can be vented; misconceptions can be corrected; and solutions to problems can be developed.

It should be asserted, however, that the potential disadvantages associated with cost-effectiveness programs are not inevitable and can be eliminated or minimized with proper planning and implementation. Furthermore, the potential advantages of cost-effectiveness in nursing far outweigh any disadvantages. The important point is that both sides must be presented, along with strong evidence suggesting that the potential disadvantages can be dealt with effectively and supporting the value and use of the potential advantages to nursing.

A fourth message characteristic found to be important in causing attitude change involves the simple repetition of the basic message. Research has shown that repetition of persuasive messages can result in significant attitudinal improvements. Repetition can occur within the content of a single message; that is, repeating the basic theme throughout the message. Repetition can also occur when the same message is repeated at different occasions. In both cases, the results are similar and repetition improves attitudes.

Efforts to improve nursing attitudes should capitalize on this simple principle and should frequently repeat the underlying theme that cost-effectiveness is useful and desirable during the delivery of a persuasive message or training session. In addition, the same basic message should be presented repeatedly through various media. For example, these might include (1) bulletin board messages, (2) organizational newsletter articles, (3) correspondence from top administrators, and (4) repetition of the message in unit meetings. The end goal is multiple exposures to the same message that should enhance attitudinal improvement.

Communicator Characteristics

The success of efforts to influence attitudes often hinges on important characteristics of the individual(s) actually presenting the persuasive communication. Research in this area has identified several critical factors that are summarized in the box, Important Communicator Characteristics in Attitude Improvement.

The first important communicator characteristic is physical attractiveness. Research has shown that greater attitude change occurs when a persuasive message is delivered by an attractive as opposed to unattractive person. Physical attractiveness increases personal liking and perceptions of competence, thus facilitating the persuasive process. Capitalizing on this phenomenon, programs to improve nursing attitudes should use a physically attractive spokesperson, if at all possible.

Second, it is highly desirable that individuals in a target group perceive the speaker as sharing some common characteris-

---

**IMPORTANT COMMUNICATOR CHARACTERISTICS
IN ATTITUDE IMPROVEMENT**

---

   1. Physical attractiveness
   2. Perceived similarity
   3. Credibility
   4. Presentational style

tic or bond. When the speaker is perceived as similar to the group on important dimensions, the prospects for successful persuasion are improved significantly. Individuals who differ greatly from the group that they are addressing are often perceived as outsiders, with little insight into the special problems of the group or sensitivity to the group's concerns.

Applications of this basic principle to programs designed to improve nursing attitudes are straightforward. Presenters should be individuals with a background, in terms of education and experience, in nursing. The use of nurses as presenters will increase the likelihood that the message content is viewed as accurate, relevant, and appropriate for nurses. A cost-effectiveness program presented by hospital administrators, productivity experts, accountants, or other business experts will not be as effective in bringing about attitudinal changes. The active involvement of nurses in communicating the basic message is absolutely essential.

The third, and perhaps most important characteristic of an effective communicator is perceived credibility. Research clearly demonstrates that messages delivered by credible as opposed to noncredible sources result in significantly more attitudinal change.

A speaker's credibility seems to depend on two critical components: perceived expertise and the lack of personal involvement or interdependence with the target group. The most persuasive communicators are those with highly perceived expertise, possessing special credentials, background, or experience that provide them with expert status. In addition, persuasiveness is enhanced by the perception that the speaker has nothing to gain personally from the situation and will not benefit from any outcomes. The combination of these two factors, perceived expertise and independence from the immediate situation, will significantly increase the amount of attitude change possible from a persuasive communication. Interestingly, these two factors also explain in large measure why external consultants are often required to implement attitude change programs within organizations.

Knowledge of these research findings should be taken into account when selecting individuals to present a program designed to improve nursing attitudes. The ideal candidate is someone who has well established expert status and who possesses special qualifications in cost-effectiveness. Furthermore, the presenter should be chosen from outside the organization to ensure independence and objectivity. Utilizing internal presenters with little perceived expertise will generally be ineffective in bringing about attitude change.

The fourth and last important communicator characteristic is the presentational style employed. Research has shown that maximum persuasiveness and attitude change can be achieved by using a smooth, fluent, friendly, and humorous presentational style. Such an approach increases personal liking for the speaker and enhances the acceptability and potency of the message. Stiff, formal, regimented, humorless presentational styles only serve to alienate an audience and are thus counterproductive in terms of inducing attitude change.

Speakers attempting to improve nursing attitudes toward cost-effectiveness would be well advised to follow these simple guidelines. The attitude change process can be facilitated by speakers who use the appropriate presentational style.

The importance of speaker characteristics in the communication process was ingeniously illustrated by Naftulin, Ware, and Donnelly.[13] In this study, a carefully scripted seminar presentation was delivered to three separate professional audiences by a distinguished-looking, physically attractive, older gentleman with an impressive vita (high expert status). His presentational style was smooth, punctuated with humor, and animated. Postsession evaluations of his presentation were uniformly positive.

Surprisingly, the actual content of his remarks was nonsensical. The script had been deliberately prepared so as to be illogical and utterly meaningless. "Dr. Fox" was a professional actor with no expertise whatsoever in the subject area. However, by virtue of his appearance, style, and perceived credibility, he was able to "seduce" a fairly sophisticated professional audience into believing that something positive, interesting, insightful, and useful had been presented.

The results of this fascinating study underscore the vital importance of speaker characteristics in the success of the communication process. These factors should be carefully considered in developing a comprehensive strategy to improve nursing attitudes toward cost-effectiveness.

Perceived Outcome Factors

Attitude change can be aided significantly by the presence of certain perceived outcomes associated with the change process. Research in this area has identified four such factors that exert a positive influence on attitude change. They are listed in the box, Important Perceived Outcome Factors in Attitude Improvement.

The first factor, participative decision making (PDM) has received a great deal of research attention. Conceptually, it is argued that people will be more receptive to the attitude change process if they are given the opportunity to realistically participate in that process and the decision making involved.

Research indicates that PDM results in less resistance to change, more acceptance of the change process, greater commitment to the process, higher levels of satisfaction, and increased attitude improvement. Most people exhibit a strong preference for participating in making important decisions that affect their work. Participation and active involvement allow for perceived ownership of the change process and lead consequently to the development of more positive attitudes, as well as supportive behaviors.

Within the nursing profession, it can be emphatically asserted that any program to improve attitudes toward cost-effectiveness should include the active participation and involvement of nurses in the target organization. Nurses should be involved at all levels of decision making and should provide input regarding program content, methods, and implementation. Attitudes toward cost-effectiveness can be substantially improved by including nurses in this process.

A specific strategy that works well is the formation of a nursing advisory council or committee to study the issue of cost-effectiveness and make policy and action recommendations. Council members are encouraged to solicit input from all staff

---

IMPORTANT PERCEIVED OUTCOME FACTORS IN ATTITUDE IMPROVEMENT

1. Participation in decision making
2. Organizational reward structure
3. Peer support and pressure
4. Fear arousal/reduction

---

members and thus the final report should realistically reflect the nursing perspective.

This basic approach was used with great success in the Methodist Hospitals of Northwest Indiana. The nursing administration recognized the need to address the cost-effectiveness problem and develop timely and effective solutions. The first step in their approach involved forming an advisory council, consisting of staff nurses, head nurses, nurse administrators, nurse academicians, and an outside management consultant, to study the hospital's problems and recommend solutions. The theme of this entire effort was "nursing-based solutions to nursing problems." Once critical problem areas had been identified, solutions were developed and communicated to staff nurses in the form of a successful 1-day seminar. Getting nurses involved in the problem solving and decision making necessary to effectively address the cost-effectiveness issue proved to be an excellent means of improving attitudes toward this issue.

A second important outcome factor revolves around the organizational reward structure. This topic is covered in more depth in Chapter 13. For purposes of the present discussion, the organizational reward structure can be viewed as having a significant impact on the development of positive attitudes toward cost-effectiveness in nursing. Organizational rewards for appropriate cost-effectiveness behaviors can result not only in more frequent exhibition of these behaviors, but also in the development of more favorable attitudes toward cost-effectiveness.

Recall that within the Fishbein and Ajzen model, attitudes are formed on the basis of one's beliefs about the particular object or topic. In terms of this model, if nurses believe that active involvement and participation will lead to desirable personal rewards from the organization, not only will they develop more positive attitudes, but they will also perform better. Thus, it is essential that nursing administrators formulate potent reward structures that recognize and reinforce cost-effective behaviors. Beliefs that cost-effectiveness will lead to valued personal rewards will result in significantly more favorable attitudes.

Similarly, a lack of participation and compliance with a cost-effectiveness program should lead directly to undesirable organizational outcomes. Thus, nurses who fail to develop appropriately positive attitudes and behaviors should receive progressively stronger organizational sanctions. For most nurses, providing rewards for cost-effectiveness behaviors will result in active program participation and significant improvements in attitudes and behavior. Sanctions should only rarely be necessary to induce involvement and compliance.

One of the basic purposes of the organization reward structure should be to influence beliefs about the consequences of cost-effective behaviors. The combination of rewards for appropriate behaviors and sanctions for inappropriate behaviors can have a tremendous impact on both attitudes and actual performance. The specific types of rewards and sanctions available are discussed in Chapter 13. Nursing administrators should not overlook the potency and use of the organizational reward structure in promoting positive attitudes toward cost-effectiveness and appropriate performance behavior.

A third important outcome factor is peer support and pressure. Research in organizational psychology has documented the importance of peer groups in influencing member attitudes, values, and behaviors at work. The desire to belong to one's work group as a member in good standing is frequently so strong that most individuals will readily conform to what they perceive as the accepted group norm.

Attempts to change attitudes and behaviors in organizations are most successful when the powerful influences of the peer group are activated in support of the program. The development and maintenance of positive attitudes and behaviors must be viewed as a group responsibility, shared equally by all members. When this is accomplished, the peer group can function to provide critical support for appropriate attitudes and behaviors, as well as potent pressures on members who deviate from the norm.

Programs to improve nursing attitudes toward cost-effectiveness should explicitly address the work group as an essential ingredient for success. The responsibility for fostering appropriate attitudes and behaviors should be placed on the work group. In order to encourage this process, nursing administrators can develop compensation systems in which the work group or nursing unit as a whole is rewarded for the attainment of cost-effectiveness objectives. This can function as a powerful incentive for the group to develop and enforce appropriate attitudes and behaviors in all members.

Finally, the fourth outcome factor that can be used to foster more positive attitudes toward cost-effectiveness involves mild fear arousal and reduction. Use of this approach requires careful attention to ensure that no exaggerated claims are made, resulting in extreme fear arousal and unnecessary distress. Social psychological research has confirmed that mild fear arousal can facilitate the attitude change process, whereas the arousal of more extreme fear is generally counterproductive.

The dynamics of this process are relatively straightforward. Recall that attitudes are based on beliefs and consider this simple illustration. If a person believes that the absence of a particular program will lead to something negative and that the presence of the program will lead to something positive, research findings and logic suggest that a favorable attitude toward the program will develop.

In the health care industry, dramatic statistics are available documenting the financial plight of many institutions and the trends that continue to exert cost pressures, such as declining admissions, reductions in length of stay, increased out-patient procedures. It can be reasonably argued that failure to respond to these powerful pressures can result in some negative outcomes, such as reductions in staff, hours worked, salary, and support resources and lead ultimately to the closing of the hospital. These outcomes are personal, real, and undesirable to most individuals. It is certainly understandable that nurses would be worried and fearful about the possibility of these events happening to their hospital and to them personally. Failure to develop and implement an effective cost control program can significantly increase the likelihood of these events occurring. Arousing mild feelings of fear in this realistic manner can be expected to enhance the development of positive attitudes toward cost-effectiveness programs, which can be viewed as instrumental in avoiding the undesirable outcomes.

The uncertainties and fears of nurses can be reduced by showing that cost-effectiveness programs can increase the probability that the hospital will remain in business, that salaries, hours, and support resources will not be cut, and that jobs will not be lost. No guarantees are possible, but those hospitals that rigorously adopt cost-effectiveness programs stand a far greater chance of survival than those that do not.

Furthermore, health care is an essential service that must be provided in our society. There will always be a need and a market for hospitals and nursing care. However, given the new competitive and financial pressures, it is predicted that many hospitals will be merged, bought-out, or bankrupt within the next decade. The successful hospitals will be those that take concerted action to control costs.

Cost-effectiveness in nursing has become a vital survival issue. An inability or unwillingness to develop positive attitudes and effective behaviors will increase the probability of organizational failure and will accelerate that process. On the other hand, the proactive formulation of favorable attitudes and cost control strategies will increase the likelihood of organizational success and continued satisfying employment.

Presenting the basic facts of the situation in this manner will serve to both arouse and hopefully reduce uncertainties and fears among nurses. The final result of the process should be the development of more positive attitudes toward cost-effectiveness. Several useful strategies to change and improve attitudes have been discussed in this chapter. As mentioned earlier, the most effective attitudinal improvement programs are those that use as many of these powerful techniques as possible.

The feasibility of successfully developing and implementing such an attitudinal improvement program was demonstrated in a study conducted by Blaney and Hobson.[10] A combination of attitudinal change strategies was shown to result in a significant improvement in nursing attitudes toward cost-effectiveness, as measured by the Blaney/Hobson Nursing Attitude Scale. The success of this effort will hopefully encourage nursing administrators to formulate similar programs to deal effectively with less-than-positive nursing attitudes in this critical area.

SUMMARY AND CONCLUSIONS

1. Given the importance and prominence of cost-effectiveness in health care, it is safe to assume that most nurses have developed strong feelings and attitudes about this issue. For

various reasons, these attitudes are, in many cases, less than positive.

2. The well-established causal link between attitudes and behavior suggests that attempts to improve the cost-effectiveness of nursing behaviors should be preceded by an assessment of the prevailing nursing attitude toward this issue. If attitudes are significantly negative, corrective strategies are necessary prior to proceeding with behavioral improvement programs.

3. The widely accepted Fishbein and Ajzen model of the attitude process postulates the following causal sequence: beliefs → attitudes → behavioral intentions → actual behaviors. This model has received consistent research support and underscores the important relationship between attitudes and behavior.

4. The Blaney/Hobson Nursing Attitude Scale is a newly developed measure of attitude toward cost-effectiveness in nursing. In rigorous research tests, it has demonstrated strong reliability and validity. Scores are positively related to cost-effective behaviors and tend to increase as one advances in nursing management/administrative positions. The scale is recommended for use in assessing the prevailing nursing attitude toward cost-effectiveness prior to initiating a program to improve behaviors.

5. The following factors have been found to increase the efficacy of a message designed to improve attitudes: (1) factual, complete, relevant, and current information, (2) simple, well-organized structure, (3) the presentation of both advantages and disadvantages associated with a particular issue, and (4) frequent repetition of the basic theme.

6. Certain communicator characteristics have been shown to increase the impact of an attitude change message. Among the more important of these are (1) physical attractiveness, (2) perceived similarity, (3) credibility (a combination of perceived expertise and lack of interdependence), and (4) a smooth, flowing, friendly, and humorous presentational style.

7. Research has shown that attitude change is facilitated by the following outcome factors: (1) allowing for active involvement and participation in decision making, (2) an organizational reward structure that recognizes and reinforces cost-effective nursing behaviors, (3) peer support and pressure to engage in cost-effective behaviors, and (4) the arousal of mild fear associated with failure to implement cost-effective behaviors and the subsequent reduction of that fear as a function of practicing the required behaviors.

Questions for Reflection and Discussion

1. Do you agree with the statement that it is essential for nurses to have a positive attitude towards cost-effectiveness? Give reasons for your answer.

2. Do you feel that the Fishbein and Ajzen model is an accurate and useful conceptualization of the attitude process?

3. Based on your experience, are people's attitudes generally related to their behavior?

4. How did you score on the Blaney/Hobson Nursing Attitude Scale and do you think this is an accurate measure of your own feelings about this issue?

5. What major beliefs about cost-effectiveness in nursing is your attitude based on?

6. What is the prevailing attitude toward cost-effectiveness among the nurses you know? What are some of the major underlying causes of this attitude?

7. What are the advantages and disadvantages of using the Blaney/Hobson Nursing Attitude Scale as a screening device in hiring nurses?

8. Of the various attitude change strategies discussed in the chapter, which do you think would be most effective in improving nursing attitudes toward cost-effectiveness? Give reasons for your answer.

REFERENCES

1. Cialdini RB, Petty RE, Cacioppo JT: Attitude and attitude change. Am Rev Psychol 32:357–404, 1981
2. Allport GW: Attitudes. In Murchinson C (ed): A Handbook of Social Psychology. Worchester, MA, Clark University Press, 1935
3. Ajzen I, Fishbein M: Attitude–behavior relations: A theoretical analysis and review of empirical research. Psychol Bull 84:888–918, 1977
4. Ajzen I, Fishbein M: Understanding Attitudes and Predicting Social Behavior. Englewood Cliffs, NJ, Prentice–Hall, 1980
5. Cooper J, Croyle RT: Attitudes and attitude change. Ann Rev Psychol 35:395–426, 1984
6. Oskamp S: Attitudes and opinions. Englewood Cliffs, NJ, Prentice–Hall, 1977
7. Fishbein M, Ajzen I: Belief, Attitude, Intention, and Behavior: An Introduction to Theory and Research. Reading, MA, Addison–Wesley, 1975
8. Likert RA: A technique for measurement of attitudes. Arch Psychol No. 140, 1932
9. Nunnally J: Psychometric Theory, 2nd ed. New York, McGraw–Hill, 1978

10. Blaney DR, Hobson CJ: Development and psychometric analysis of a scale to measure attitude toward cost-effectiveness in nursing. In Waltz CF, Strickland OL (eds): Measurement of Nursing Outcomes. New York, Springer (in press)
11. Baron RA, Byrne D: Social Psychology: Understanding Human Interaction, 4th ed. Boston, Allyn and Bacon, 1984
12. Rajecki DW: Attitudes: Themes and Advances. Sunderland, MA, Sinauer Associates, 1982
13. Naftulin DH, Ware JE, Jr, Donnelly FA: The Doctor Fox lecture: A paradigm of educational seduction. J Med Educ 48:630–635, 1973

5

Motivating Desired New Behaviors Through Incentives' Analysis

NURSES WILL be required to learn, master, and practice new, more cost-effective methods of providing patient care in order to respond successfully to the emerging challenges in health care. These required performance improvements are primarily a function of two major components: motivation and ability. Nurses must be motivated properly to learn, master, and practice the skills necessary to improve the cost-effectiveness of the patient care process. They must also be provided with opportunities to improve their ability to provide cost-effective care by learning new skills, procedures, and techniques.

Both motivation and ability are critical in determining the ultimate level and success of nursing performance. Motivational issues are dealt with in Part 1 of this book while several important ability dimensions are specifically addressed in Part 2. The purpose of the present chapter is to focus explicitly on motivation and its role as a determinant of nursing performance.

The concept of motivation is defined and a comprehensive theoretical framework is introduced and explained. Next, the various types of incentives and reward programs are discussed, followed by an analysis of the current situation in nursing, in terms of the motivational climate and available incentives. Finally, a systematic prescription for nursing action is presented.

MOTIVATION — DEFINITION OF A CONCEPT

Within the context of behavior in organizations, motivation can be defined as the set of psychological processes that energize a person's behavior, direct it toward attaining some goal, and sustain it over time. Motivation thus deals with three critical questions about human behavior: (1) what initially activates or energizes a person's behavior, (2) what gives behavioral direction, and (3) what sustains behavior or causes it to persist over time. The corresponding motivational questions facing nurse managers are given in Table 5-1.

Successful motivational programs must first begin by asking the correct questions. Systematic and comprehensive answers to the three nursing questions listed in Table 5-1 will provide a useful framework for motivating nurses. Finding workable answers to these questions represents a major challenge for all nurse managers. The remaining material in this chapter is intended to help nurse managers to begin to formulate informed answers and strategies to effectively approach these critical questions.

Before proceeding to the next section, it is useful to make a distinction between two basic types of motivation — intrinsic and extrinsic. Deci defines intrinsic motivation as the motivation to

Table 5-1.   Basic Motivational Questions Facing Nurse Managers

Basic Motivational Questions	*Corresponding Nursing Questions*
1. What initially activates or energizes behavior?	1. What can be done to get nurses excited about improving the cost-effectiveness of patient care?
2. What gives behavior direction?	2. What can be done to encourage nurses to learn and use new cost-effective practices?
3. What causes behavior to persist over time?	3. What can be done to ensure that new cost-effective practices continue to be used over time?

engage in an activity for which there is no apparent reward except the activity itself,[1] in other words, the individual is motivated simply by performing the activity. Extrinsic motivation, on the other hand, involves engaging in an activity for the material outcomes that it brings.

This distinction can be important in the work environment. People who are intrinsically motivated are those who freely, willingly, and enthusiastically perform a task because they want to. The very act of performing the activity is in some way motivating and satisfying, leading to such feelings as accomplishment, excitement, self-respect, or pride. For example, a nurse might spend a great deal of time trying to console a pediatric patient who is crying. The nurse is motivated intrinsically to do this and needs no additional incentive, because helping the child is rewarding.

A person who is motivated extrinsically performs tasks, not because they like to, but because they feel that they must, in order to obtain desired material outcomes. The task to them is simply a means to an end.

The implications of the intrinsic/extrinsic difference are probably obvious. People work better and harder when they are motivated intrinsically, performing a task because they want to, not because they have to. Consequently, nurse managers would be well advised to try to develop and nurture intrinsic motivation among their staff, with respect to the new requirements for enhanced cost-effectiveness. Intrinsically motivated nurses will implement and use cost-effective care strategies more effectively.

Although there is no simple or straightforward formula for developing intrinsic motivation, there are general guidelines that can be helpful in this regard that are discussed throughout the chapter. Successfully fostering intrinsic motivation requires a great deal of time and effort from the manager. However, it can be cogently argued that the reward, in terms of improved performance, is well worth the effort.

THEORETICAL FRAMEWORK AND HOW TO USE IT

Several popular comprehensive theories of human motivation include Maslow's Need Hierarchy, Herzberg's Two Factor Theory, and McGregor's Theory X–Theory Y. Unfortunately, the results are disappointing when these well-known theories are subjected to rigorous research tests. Hobson, Meade, and Soverly briefly reviewed the research summaries available for each of these three approaches and found that years of testing have failed to generate any consistent support for their accuracy or usefulness in explaining the process of human motivation.[2]

If these popular theories do not work well, what does? Fortunately, one approach has generated considerable research support and is widely accepted as the best comprehensive theory of work motivation presently available.[3-5] It is known as *expectance theory* and was first introduced by Vroom.[6]

Since its introduction, a great deal of research has been conducted to test the theory and its usefulness in explaining and predicting human behavior. Miner reviewed this research and concluded that the approach has consistently been able to explain motivation in work settings, at levels far greater than those possible with other theories.[5] Ivancevich and Matteson noted, with rare exceptions, that over 50 studies testing the theory have demonstrated strong support.[4]

Expectancy theory, however, is not a perfect theory of motivation and does not work with everyone. Human behavior is so diverse and complex that one single theory cannot be expected to explain everything. Nevertheless, given the current state of knowledge regarding motivation in organizations, it is the best available theory and thus can serve as a useful framework for evaluating motivational issues in nursing.

At first glance, Vroom's theory is somewhat imposing and appears to be complex and difficult to understand. Subsequent revisions of the theory often added further to this perceived complexity and difficulty. Nevertheless, the basic components of this approach are simple and its implications for practice are straightforward.

The theory represents a cognitive approach to motivation. Vroom asserted that motivation is based on the way people perceive and think about the world around them.[6] Thus, perceptions and thoughts are the fundamental building blocks of expectancy theory.

According to Vroom, motivation to put forth a high level of effort in a particular job or task is a function of two basic components: (1) the person's subjective belief that if they try hard, they can be successful, and (2) the person's perception that successful performance will lead to valued outcomes. These two factors are depicted in Figure 5-1.

Consider these two components from a personal perspective. If someone wants you to really try hard and exert a great deal of effort on a particular task, they must first convince you of two things: (1) that you can succeed at the task if you try hard; that is, you have all of the required skills and abilities, and (2) that success on the task will be followed by valued outcomes. If they can convince you of these two conditions, there is a strong probability that you will try hard and exert a great deal of effort. Of course, not everyone will respond as predicted, but most people will.

To underscore the impact of the aforementioned two factors on human motivation, consider what would occur in their absence. For example — would you try hard and exert effort on a particular task if you knew that you could not possibly be successful because you lack certain essential skills or abilities? Most people would respond negatively. In the second case, would you try hard and exert effort in order to be successful on a task if you perceived that there were no rewards or incentives associated with success (in fact, you might simply be exhausted from trying so hard)? Again, usually the answer is negative. Certainly, over an extended time, most people will not continue to exert a high level of effort unless they believe that they can be successful and that positive outcomes will follow.

Hopefully, the simplicity of the basic components of the theory is evident. Good theories do not necessarily need to be complicated. These fundamental concepts can be powerful when applied in the work environment to motivate staff members. The steps in the process of applying expectancy theory are straightforward and considered commonsensical by many people. Significant improvements in staff performance can result from consist-

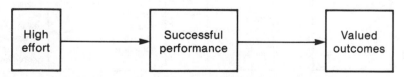

FIGURE 5-1. *The basic operation of expectancy theory.*

ently following these steps and developing the necessary motivational framework.

An overview of the four basic steps involved in using expectancy theory is provided in Figure 5-2. These steps are briefly introduced in this section and are then more fully discussed in the section entitled "A Prescription for Nursing Action."

The first step consists of clearly specifying performance expectations and outcomes. In order to effectively motivate someone, the individual must first know exactly what is expected of her and what she is supposed to do. Furthermore, it is also desirable to clarify reward and punishment contingencies; in other words, what positive outcomes are associated with good performance and what negative ones are associated with poor performance. Managers should clearly establish these performance–outcome relationships in order to communicate to staff members the consequences associated with their performance behaviors.

The second step in the motivational process includes properly training staff members and providing them with the support necessary for success. The knowledge, skills, and abilities required for effective performance should be identified by the manager and then incorporated into training programs for staff members. Remember, trying hard or exerting a great deal of effort is contingent on the belief that one can be successful at the task. Thus, a person without the necessary knowledge, skills, or abilities will not be motivated to try hard. Managers must also do everything within their power to provide staff members with the resources needed for effectiveness in terms of equipment, funding, staffing, and so forth.

The third step in the process entails accurately measuring performance behaviors. This topic is the focus of attention in Chapter 6. Managers must develop objective, accurate, and com-

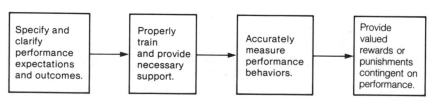

FIGURE 5-2. *Four steps in motivating staff.*

prehensive systems to measure performance in order to be able to identify good and poor performers. Rewards and punishments cannot be dispensed properly without an accurate method of measuring job performance. Motivation to try hard is partly a function of the perceived rewards associated with success. The entire process will be disrupted if a successful performance cannot be validly measured.

The fourth and final step in the expectancy theory approach involves actually dispensing rewards and punishments contingent on performance levels. Rewards promised for good performance in step one should be delivered. Failure to follow through and provide promised rewards can be disastrous and can ruin staff motivation; likewise, sanctions and disciplinary actions promised for poor performance must also be delivered. Failure to act as stated will substantially weaken a manager's ability to motivate her staff.

Significant improvements in staff motivation can result from following this relatively simple and straightforward set of four steps. The time and effort required to develop a structured motivation system like this is well worth the effort and will immeasurably increase both personal and organizational effectiveness.

TYPES OF REWARD PROGRAMS AND INCENTIVES

Recall that, according to Vroom, a person's motivation to try hard and put forth a great deal of effort is a function of two factors: (1) her belief that by trying hard she can be successful, and (2) her perceptions concerning the rewards associated with being successful. In this section, the discussion focuses on the second factor — perceived rewards or incentives. Before presenting the different types of reward programs and available incentives, five general comments concerning incentives will be made.

First, research in organizational behavior clearly demonstrates that people do respond to incentives.[7] Human behavior is guided mainly by the perceived outcomes associated with different potential courses of action. If one alternative course is expected to result in positive outcomes, and a second in negative ones, most people would clearly choose the former. Consequently, explicitly linking valued outcomes to performance can serve as a powerful motivational tool.

Second, it is well known that no two people are alike. These individual differences show up in employee preferences for various types of rewards. What is desirable, satisfying, and rewarding to one person may be totally unimportant, or even offensive, to another person. For example, additional autonomy and decision-making authority could be viewed favorably by one staff member and could thus be used as an incentive or reward for good performance. Another person, however, might view the same situation in a negative manner, wishing to avoid additional autonomy and authority. The message to managers is clear: staff members have different values and should ideally be rewarded accordingly.

Third, it is important to keep in mind that people like to regard themselves as winners. Peters and Waterman have observed that the best managed companies in the United States design their incentive systems so that most of their employees are rewarded and thus feel like winners.[8] People who feel good about themselves and believe that they are winners tend to work better and harder than others and also to be more satisfied. An example of how this idea is applied in industry is illustrated in the way that IBM manages its sales staff so that 70% to 80% achieve or meet their sales quota and are appropriately recognized and rewarded. Rather than reserving rewards only for the top 10% of the sales group, IBM wants most of their sales personnel to be clearly labeled as winners. This simple yet potent insight should be borne in mind when developing incentive plans in any organization.

Fourth in this chapter, the exclusive focus is on the use of incentives or rewards as a means to motivate behavior. The necessity for punishment, sanctions, and progressive discipline in certain situations is clearly recognized and is critical to long-term success in management.[9] However, research has shown that most adult workers respond favorably to the systematic use of incentives to motivate their behavior.[10-12] For example, Hamner argued that most people who enter the work force do so willingly and have been conditioned by their parents and society to know the difference between right and wrong.[10] As mature individuals, the only technique that is needed to motivate them is the presence or absence of positively valued rewards. Thus, in most instances, managers do not need to use punishment to control behavior.

Reliance on punishment as a motivational tool is largely ineffective and dysfunctional in influencing human behavior. Wiard has argued that the use of punishment in organizations is inappropriate in most situations and rarely leads to desirable outcomes.[12] From a strictly personal perspective, how do you respond to a supervisor who uses punishment, threats, and intimidation to motivate, as opposed to using rewards and incentives?

Whereas most people respond well to the positive approach, nurse managers must recognize the importance of progression in those infrequent occasions when someone deliberately and repeatedly performs poorly or resists authority. The ramifications of failing to punish in such situations are disastrous. Discipline is compromised and one's ability to manage, not only the problem employee, but also others, is severely impaired.

As expectancy theory indicates, punishment should be clearly linked to poor performance and then delivered as promised, using the notion of progressive discipline. In other words, continued occurrences of poor performance should result in progressively more severe punishments, ultimately leading to discharge for chronically poor workers.

Again, it should be emphasized, that most people will respond favorably to the exclusive use of incentives. However, effectiveness as a nurse manager necessitates the capacity to punish, although managers are only infrequently required to exercise this capacity.

The fifth and final general point involves the fundamental issue that every nurse manager must address concerning the use of incentives — "What do I control that my staff members value?" Systematically answering this question will result in the formulation of a "reward inventory," consisting of specific incentives that can be used to develop an effective motivational program. This can often be a useful exercise for nurse managers, and most are surprised at the length of the list of valued outcomes over which they exercise direct and immediate control.

Only a person's imagination limits the types of performance incentives that can be developed and used. If you have problems identifying items for your reward inventory, simply ask your staff members what you could do for them. Their responses will indicate what you control that they value and provide you with critical information for the development of a successful program.

There is nearly an infinite variety of ways to structure reward programs in organizations. However, it is useful to consider such programs as consisting of three basic types: (1) individual, (2) group, and (3) organization-wide. Each of these has its own advantages and disadvantages. Furthermore, the effectiveness of each basic type depends on the situation in which it is used. The challenge to nurse managers is to develop incentive programs that work effectively within the parameters and constraints of their particular organization.

Individual Reward Programs

Individual reward programs are structured to provide incentives directly to single employees, based on their own performance. Such programs are only appropriate when an employee's personal performance or contribution can be measured accurately. Otherwise, it is impossible to base rewards on individual performance. It is also difficult to accurately assess the unique contribution of a single person in many team or group activities; thus, individual rewards would not be appropriate in these settings.

The major advantage of individual reward programs is the explicit, clear-cut linkage between a person's performance and her own reward. Increased effort and performance lead directly to a corresponding increase in rewards. Individual motivation is maximized in such situations. It is also possible to stimulate healthy, productive competition among workers in an organization who are striving to be the best and achieve the largest reward.

Individual reward programs also have several potentially serious disadvantages. For example, unhealthy and dysfunctional competition can arise between employees in the same group. Instead of cooperating and working together, people compete against each other and divisive conflicts can result. Thus, individual rewards can act to discourage cooperation and team work among fellow employees. This is especially problematic when groups work closely together; when they are highly interdependent; and when individual contributions cannot be measured easily or accurately.

Consider the following actual example from an industrial facility as an example of the misuse of individual rewards. A crew of five workers had established a facility-wide production record. One of the crew members was designated as the operator and generally coordinated the activities of the entire crew. However, everyone was absolutely essential in the production process and worked closely together. The entire process stopped if one person failed to do her job.

Management in this particular organization wanted to reward this fine effort in establishing a new production record. They chose to provide the operator with a drive-in pass, which would allow him to park next to the facility and thus to avoid parking in an off-site parking area and walking to the facility. The other four crew members received verbal congratulations only.

The impact of this short-sighted strategy was immediate and pronounced. Crew productivity fell sharply and internal dissention increased dramatically. After only 1 month, the operator disgustedly returned the drive-in pass in an attempt to restore the harmony and team work that had previously existed. The managers had made a serious mistake in using individual rewards with a highly interdependent group and they paid dearly for it.

Group Reward Programs

The second basic type of reward program involves providing performance incentives to entire work groups as opposed to individual employees. Rewards are contingent on the performance level achieved by the group as a whole. These programs are most appropriate when employees are highly interdependent and work closely together as a team. In such situations, it is often difficult or impossible to accurately measure the unique contribution of individual group members. For example, in the industrial setting involving the five person crew described earlier, group rewards would clearly have been more appropriate.

Major potential advantages of group-based reward programs include (1) promoting intragroup cooperation and cohesion, (2) mobilizing peer pressure to help motivate poorly performing group members, and (3) healthy, productive intergroup competition. On the other hand, providing group rewards can in some situations act to discourage good workers from trying hard and performing well, given that everyone receives the same incentive. The good performer might feel that she is undercompensated for the work that she does compared to others, whereas poor performers are overcompensated. Perceived equity of reward systems is critical to program success.[13,14] Consequently, it is important that top performers perceive that their rewards are higher than those given to poor performers. Individual motivation suffers when serious inequity exists. Thus, one important drawback of group rewards is the potential for perceived reward inequity.

Another related disadvantage of group reward programs is the lack of a direct, clear-cut relationship between a person's performance and the reward that she receives. It is unfortunately not always the case that the better one performs, the more one is rewarded. Some individuals respond to situations such as this by engaging in social loafing, whereby they rely on others to work hard and earn the rewards for the group as a whole. Finally, group-based rewards can result in unhealthy, destructive competition among groups in an organization, especially if one group's gain is another's loss.

Organization-wide Reward Programs

These types of reward programs provide incentives to all members of an organization, regardless of individual performance level. They have been most successfully used in relatively small, homogeneous, and cohesive companies. Such programs offer several potentially important advantages: (1) generating good will with all organizational employees, (2) promoting a sense of equality, community, and team spirit, and (3) facilitating intergroup cooperation.

In terms of disadvantages, organization-wide reward programs are psychologically distant from individual employees. The connection between personal performance and pay is tenuous at best. Since everyone receives the same reward, top performers are likely to view themselves as inequitably underpaid, whereas social loafing and lack of effort are rewarded. Heterogeneous companies that have many departments that differ in terms of their productivity and that pay everyone the same wages, can actually lead to resentment and conflict between departments.

Reward programs can thus be structured at any one of three levels — individual, group, or organization-wide. Each type works best in certain kinds of situations and has its own unique advantages and disadvantages. Decisions regarding what kind of reward program to use in a particular organization should be based on a thorough analysis of specific program objectives and relevant company characteristics. More information on these issues as they relate to nursing is found in the section entitled "A Prescription for Nursing Action."

Monetary Incentives

Performance incentives fall into two basic categories — monetary and nonmonetary. The monetary category includes the many ways in which to use pay as an incentive for performance. The private sector has long recognized the powerful potential of monetary rewards in motivating performance and stimulating productivity. Lawler was one of the first scholars to systematically address this issue and his book triggered a great deal of interest among American business leaders.[15]

According to Ivancevich and Matteson, the pay-for performance movement is growing in popularity as the excellent bottom-line results encourage more companies to revamp their reward systems.[4] They cite a Hay Management Consultant's survey of 600 firms which found that, although 11% of the companies presently had pay-for-performance systems, three times as many had plans to develop and implement such programs in the future.

Monetary incentive systems seem to be proliferating most rapidly in the more competitive industries. For example, in the grocery business, competition is keen, costs are rising, and profit margins are slim — a situation similar to that developing in health care. *Business Week* reported on how the A&P supermarket chain managed to successfully reduce their costs and substantially increase profits.[16] Workers were told that monetary bonuses would be paid to them for reductions in labor costs. The specific arrangements were detailed in advance — if labor costs were kept to 10% of store sales, a cash bonus equal to 1% of sales would be distributed to all employees. Further decreases in labor costs would result in corresponding increases in the bonus percentage.

Employees were thus encouraged to work harder and accomplish more in fewer hours (a common exhortation in health care these days). However, in exchange for this additional effort, they were promised, and actually received, significant cash bonuses.

As a result of this program, A&P has increased its operating profit since 1984 by 81% and its stock value has doubled in price to $24.00. Their approach has been an overwhelming success and clearly demonstrates the potential use of carefully constructed monetary incentive systems in improving performance and productivity.

A wide variety of incentive programs involving monetary rewards has been developed and used in American industry. In this section, the major program types are presented and discussed at the three levels introduced earlier — individual, group, and organization-wide. The presentation is restricted to approaches that are based directly or indirectly on performance and are designed to improve productivity levels. An overview of the specific strategies is found in the box, Basic Types of Monetary Incentives.

At the individual level, the most basic form of monetary incentive is the piece rate system, in which a worker is paid a certain amount for each unit produced. The relationship between performance and reward is perfect — the more you produce, the more reward you receive. Piece rate pay plans can be used successfully in any situation where individual performance can be measured in terms of the number of items produced.

The second type of individual program is the merit pay increase; in other words, an individual's level of performance over a period of time (usually 1 year) forms the basis for determining a salary increase. The better a person performs, the higher her raise will be during the following year. Merit salary increases are

---

BASIC TYPES OF MONETARY INCENTIVES

1. *Individual incentives*
   - Piece rate
   - Merit pay
   - Merit bonus
   - Salary *vs* hourly wage

2. *Group or departmental incentives*
   - Gain sharing

3. *Organizational incentives*
   - Profit sharing
   - Stock ownership

---

used widely in business and industry as a means of rewarding and motivating performance. This approach serves to permanently increase a person's base salary level and thus represents a long-term commitment by the organization.

On the other hand, merit bonuses (the third type of individual program) involve the payment of a one-time cash amount, based on performance level. The bonus does not serve to increase the person's base salary level in future years and consequently represents a more cost-effective way to reward performance than using merit salary increases.

The fourth and final monetary incentive program for individuals involves the payment of salaries as opposed to hourly wages. The Japanese have pioneered the use of this motivational technique as a means both of enhancing productivity and improving employee relations. The following advantages are often associated with all-salaried work forces: (1) the divisions and conflicts between management and employees are minimized, (2) worker trust and commitment are increased, (3) the dysfunctional "employee mentality" is reduced significantly, and (4) overall performance and productivity can be improved dramatically.

At the group or departmental level, the generic term for monetary incentive programs is *gain sharing*. This typically involves paying a one-time bonus to all members of a work group, based on overall performance or productivity. Specific target measures must first be carefully defined and then explicitly linked to the available bonus. The A&P example cited earlier illustrates a type of gain-sharing program. Store employees were given a bonus equivalent to 1% of store sales if labor costs were held to 10% total sales. Thus, each employee benefited equally if the overall cost containment objective was met.

Finally, there are two basic types of organization-wide monetary incentive programs: profit sharing and stock ownership. Profit sharing involves distributing some agreed on percentage of a company's profits to all employees. This can be accomplished either by giving everyone the same dollar amount or by basing payment on the individual's salary level or hourly rate. Profit sharing plans have proliferated rapidly in the United States and have become a major issue in collective bargaining contracts. The logic of such plans is compelling. By tying employee compensation to the overall profitability of the firm, individual commitment, motivation, and productivity are often improved significantly.

The second organization-wide program provides company stock to employees as a performance incentive. The dollar value of stock shares can be calculated easily in terms of the stock's current market price. Stocks also typically pay quarterly dividends. In addition to the monetary value, rewarding employees with company stock makes them partial owners of the company and thus more committed to the company's success and willing to work hard. Progressive organizations in the United States have long used stock ownership plans as an excellent means of motivating their work force and of building loyalty and commitment.

Nonmonetary Incentives

Various nonmonetary incentive programs have been developed successfully and have been used to improve worker motivation and performance. Within the field of organizational behavior, a major focus of recent research has been on the topic of job design — how to structure jobs and work environments using nonmonetary components to increase employee motivation, satisfaction, and performance. The most widely accepted theory of job design is the Job Characteristics Model, originally developed by Hackman and Oldham.[17,18] Their approach is based on the assumption that critical task characteristics and nonmonetary incentives are the keys to understanding individual work motivation. Findings generated from this theory and other related research have significantly expanded the knowledge base concerning nonmonetary rewards and their impact on behavior.

Before discussing the various types of nonmonetary rewards, it is useful to first address important general aspects that apply to all of them. Nonmonetary rewards are typically considered and dispensed at the level of the individual employee and not at the work group or organization-wide level. Studies have repeatedly shown that workers in the United States often place a higher value on nonmonetary as opposed to monetary rewards. Consequently, a well-formulated program consisting of nonmonetary incentives can represent a potent and cost-effective means of motivating staff.

Nonmonetary rewards, in comparison to monetary ones, have a significantly greater impact on intrinsic motivation; that is, an individual's desire to do a good job because she "wants to," not because she "has to." Finally, nonmonetary rewards are typically under the direct and immediate control of the supervisor. This can provide managers with a source of potentially powerful incentives to use in motivating staff members.

A listing of the major nonmonetary incentives that have been successfully developed and used is found in the box, Basic Types of Nonmonetary Incentives. Each is discussed briefly.

Perhaps the most important nonmonetary incentive is recognition for good work. Unfortunately, most managers do a poor job in providing positive feedback to their staff.[19] Employees universally report that they enjoy receiving genuine positive feedback from their employers and that they do not get enough of it. Managers should use this valuable information to their advantage by developing both formal and informal recognition programs as a means of motivating performance.

Opportunities for advancement and promotion also constitute an effective use of nonmonetary incentives. While promotions entail additional pay in many organizations, they can be employed effectively as a means of rewarding achievement and conferring additional status on good performers, without involving money.

Participation in decision making is highly valued by most individuals and can thus serve as a powerful nonmonetary incentive. People generally desire input into decisions affecting their work environment. This privilege to participate is under the

---

BASIC TYPES OF NONMONETARY INCENTIVES

Recognition
Advancement and promotion
Participation in decision making
Autonomy
Task rotation and skill variety
Task completion
Feeling of belonging and usefulness
Understanding and help with personal problems
Professional development opportunities
Time banking

direct control of the supervisor and can be extended to individual employees on the basis of their job performance.

Autonomy in planning and executing work activities can function for many employees as a potent motivator. Although some people prefer to be told exactly and continuously what to do, most individuals value some discretion in how they perform their jobs.

Task rotation and skill variety involve allowing individuals to work at different tasks requiring various skills. This technique is designed to overcome the boredom, lethargy, and lack of motivation often associated with performing the same routine task repeatedly. The traditional assembly line is a classic example. Most people respond favorably to some degree of change and variety in what they do at work. Thus, the supervisor can reward good performers by allowing for rotation among several different tasks.

Employees generally express a strong preference for working on a particular task from start to finish, as opposed to repetitively performing one single operation in a larger task process. For example, in the traditional assembly line, workers perform one routine operation continuously and are not afforded the opportunity to work on a task from start to finish, resulting in some whole or meaningful outcome. Managers can use this knowledge to motivate staff members by designing work tasks and projects that involve employees from start to finish, thus allowing for feelings of ownership, accomplishment, and pride.

People also like to believe that they serve a useful function at work, that they are needed, and that they are an important part of the work effort. Managers exert a powerful influence over feelings like these and can develop strategies to create and reinforce them as a means of rewarding and motivating good performance.

In addition, supervisors can serve as an important source of understanding and help for employees with personal problems. Everyone is confronted with problems at some point that affect their work performance. Understanding and help from the supervisor can not only assist the person in dealing with her problem, but can also significantly increase motivation and commitment.

Professional development opportunities are positively valued by many employees and can be used effectively by the supervisor as a means of rewarding and motivating good performers. Examples include allowing employees to attend special classes, seminars, or job-related conferences.

The last type of nonmonetary incentive is time banking. This relatively new approach holds tremendous promise as a means of motivating employees. It involves rewarding good performers with scheduled time off; in other words, employees earn paid time off as a function of performance level. Those employees meeting productivity or cost-related goals are compensated with a certain number of hours, which can be accumulated over time and taken in half-day or full-day increments. Ivancevich and Matteson note that, given the prevailing values of workers in the United States, earned time off can be an effective means of stimulating performance and productivity.[4]

In summary, a wide variety of powerful monetary and nonmonetary incentives are available for use in motivating and rewarding employees. What works best in a particular situation will depend on the manager involved, employee values, and organizational characteristics. The challenge to nurse managers is to find the combination of incentives that works best for them.

CURRENT MOTIVATION CLIMATE AND AVAILABLE INCENTIVES IN NURSING

It is widely agreed that, in order to meet the new challenges in health care, nurses must learn and master new, more cost-effective ways of providing patient care. According to Vroom, the motivation to do this is a function of two factors: (1) nurses' perceptions that by trying hard they will be able to successfully perform the required new behaviors and (2) nurses' perceptions of the outcomes associated with mastering these new behaviors.[6] In this section, the focus is on analyzing the current situation in nursing in terms of the perceived outcomes associated with cost-effectiveness. Additional motivational issues are also discussed.

Research in psychology has shown conclusively that people respond to incentives. They behave in ways that correspond to perceived rewards and punishments in their environment. It is useful to examine the current nursing situation in terms of the perceived rewards and punishments associated with cost-effective behaviors.

Extensive empirical data relevant to this issue are not available. Two sources of information, however, were used as a basis for the arguments presented here. The first source is a published article in *Nursing Life,* reporting the results of a survey dealing with DRG's and cost-related matters in nursing.[20] The second source consists of the verbal responses of nurses to two questions asked in cost-effectiveness seminars conducted by Blaney and Hobson — what do you see as the major advantage of cost-effectiveness in nursing and what do you see as the major disadvantage?

The basic concern is that if nurses perceive that cost-effectiveness leads to undesirable outcomes, they will be less than enthusiastic in learning, implementing, and using new techniques. Success in this area depends on providing nurses with positively valued rewards for cost-effective performance.

Based upon the *Nursing Life* survey and the answers to the two questions given above, staff nurses generally believe that cost-effectiveness will lead (1) directly to undesirable outcomes (*i.e.,* lower quality patient care) or (2) to the avoidance of undesirable outcomes (*i.e.,* preventing staff cuts).[20] Cost-effectiveness is only rarely perceived as resulting in positive outcomes for nursing. The outcomes commonly associated with cost-effective nursing practices are summarized in Figure 5-3.

comes with cost-effectiveness (Fig. 5-3). These include lower quality patient care, staffing cuts, increased work loads, and further budget cuts. These factors constitute powerful punish-

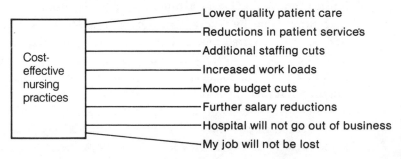

FIGURE 5-3. *Major outcomes commonly associated with cost-effective nursing practices.*

ments for most nurses and function to discourage participation in cost-effectiveness programs. For example, one nurse reported that a successful effort to reduce costs in her unit was "rewarded" by subtracting the amount saved from the budget for the following year and requested that additional cuts be made. Unfortunately, if nurses really believe that cost-effective strategies will result in undesirable outcomes, their cooperation and support will be minimal.

In some cases, nurses feel that by using cost-effective techniques, they can avoid unpleasant consequences, such as closing the hospital or losing their jobs. The term for this motivational situation is *negative reinforcement;* that is, nurses are engaging in a particular behavior only to avoid an undesirable outcome. Regrettably, few nurses perceive that cost-effectiveness will lead directly to positive outcomes.

Attempting to encourage new cost-conscious behaviors in nursing by employing punishment and negative reinforcement is unwise and ineffective. The use of positive reinforcement and rewards is clearly the preferred alternative, although rarely practiced in any systematic manner. Until this state of affairs is changed dramatically, progress in improving productivity and efficiency in nursing will be slow.

Certainly not all staff nurses feel that cost-effectiveness will result only in negative outcomes or their avoidance, but the best available data suggest that many of them do. Nurse managers are advised to ask staff members about their perceptions in this area.

There are some encouraging signs that nurses and health care managers are beginning to realize the importance of incentives to the success of cost-effectiveness programs. For instance, the *Wall Street Journal* cited a Hay Group Consultant's report indicating that executive incentive pay linked to productivity would likely be in effect at 25% to 28% of the nonprofit hospitals in the United States in 1985, up from a mere 1% in 1981.[21] Madsen and Harper have observed that some hospitals are beginning to design incentive programs that reward nursing units with the smallest number of lost charges for supplies and equipment.[22] In perhaps the most noteworthy example, Schnee, Robbins, and Robbins described a successful monetary incentive program for nurses that linked pay to productivity at the individual, nursing unit, and hospital-wide level.[23] These and other similar efforts indicate that the health care field in general and nursing in particular are beginning to fully appreciate the incentive programs in improving cost-effectiveness.

Although the identification and use of valued rewards are essential to the success of any incentive program, other issues are equally important. For example, do nurses agree as to what specific cost-effective techniques are needed? Do nurses have the necessary training in order to perform these required new behaviors? Are performance appraisal systems available to accurately measure the desired behaviors? Unfortunately, in most cases, adequate and complete answers to these critical questions have not yet been formulated. Success in motivating nurses requires that these issues be dealt with. In the next section, a systematic approach to designing incentive systems to effectively reward and motivate nurses is presented.

PRESCRIPTION FOR NURSING ACTION

In order to significantly improve the cost-effectiveness of the patient care process, nurse managers must develop, implement, and use a systematic framework for motivating their staff. Success is unlikely without competent, enthusiastic staff participation in cost-effective efforts.

Vroom's expectancy theory provides a useful model for formulating a motivational program in nursing. The theory translates into a relatively straightforward four-step process for motivating employees: (1) specify and clarify performance expectations and outcomes, (2) properly train and provide necessary support, (3) accurately measure performance behaviors, and (4) provide valued rewards/punishments contingent on performance. The practical issues involved in successfully developing, implementing, and using this approach are presented and discussed.

Step 1. Specify and clarify performance expectations and outcomes. In this first step, nurse managers must determine exactly what they expect of staff nurses, in terms of new, more cost-effective patient care practices. These expectations must be defined explicitly in behavioral terminology; in other words, what specific behaviors are to be expected of staff members. If, for example, a new inventory control system is to be introduced, what specific new practices is the nurse expected to follow? If an improved approach to patient teaching is introduced, exactly how is the nurse expected to use it? In every case, the actual behaviors involved should be identified and defined unambiguously, leaving no confusion in the nurse's mind as regarding what is expected.

A critical factor must be considered when specifying these performance expectations — the quality of performance. Nurse managers must ensure that quality expectations, not simply quantity, are clearly communicated. It is not enough to simply process a certain number of patients per shift or perform a specific set of procedures, without concern for quality. In all cases, high quality care must be a major performance objective for which nurses are rewarded.

Once new performance expectations have been clarified and cogently communicated to staff members, it is then necessary to stipulate the outcomes associated with different levels of performance. For instance, what outcomes will be provided to good performers and what will be given to poor ones? These performance – outcome contingencies must be established clearly in order to optimally motivate staff members.

It was previously asserted that most adult workers can be motivated effectively by using incentives and rewards for good performance as opposed to punishments for poor performance. This general principle also applies in most nursing settings. Therefore, the development and use of positive incentive programs will suffice to motivate most nurses to practice more cost-effective behaviors. In fact, the *Nursing Life* survey mentioned earlier revealed that 63% of those reponding felt that the use of performance incentives for nurses could make their department more cost-effective.[20] These results should convey a clear message to all nurse managers that the time for incentives is now.

Recall that incentive programs can be structured at any one of three levels — individual, group, and organization-wide. It is our strong contention that reward programs should be formulated at all three levels in order to maximally motivate individual, unit, and hospital-wide productivity and encourage cooperation and team work. The approach taken by Schnee and associates is an excellent practical example of how such programs can be developed and operated.[23]

The nurse manager is faced with a different kind of decision concerning which of the two basic types of incentives (monetary and nonmonetary) to best use in motivating staff members. In all likelihood, a combination of both types represents the best approach. Available research on the determinants of nursing job satisfaction indicates that both monetary and nonmonetary rewards are valued positively in the profession.[24,25] Consequently, both should be incorporated into comprehensive motivational programs.

Given the overriding emphasis on economic and financial considerations in health care, we firmly believe that monetary incentives must be a part of any plan to motivate staff members. Asking nurses to begin thinking and acting in a more cost-effective manner without rewarding good performance monetarily is unfair and short-sighted. Success in such endeavors requires that nursing efforts be rewarded financially. Failure to understand this important concept will substantially inhibit the effectiveness of any motivational program.

Although financial incentives are considered essential in promoting cost-effectiveness in nursing, the value of nonmonetary rewards should not be overlooked. Gordon and others have recognized the importance of creating a motivating environment for nurses, consisting primarily of nonmonetary factors.[26] The list in the box, Basic Types of Nonmonetary Incentives, should convince nurse managers that they control several powerful outcomes that their staff values, including recognition, participation in decision making, autonomy, and time banking. Managers can exert a tremendous influence on staff motivation by using these outcomes in the reward system.

Lack of recognition, for example, is a common complaint not only of workers everywhere, but also in nursing. Thus, nurse managers should not underestimate the overwhelming potential impact of positive feedback, given formally or on an informal, face-to-face basis. To illustrate the possibilities, formal recognition can be accomplished in any of the following ways: (1) prominently displaying the picture of the "Nurse of the Month" on the unit or departmental bulletin board, (2) conducting awards and recognition ceremonies at the unit, departmental, or hospital level, and (3) publishing noteworthy accomplishments in a nursing or hospital newsletter.

As mentioned earlier, most nurses should respond favorably to a positive approach, using monetary and nonmonetary incentives to encourage and reward cost-effective behaviors. However, it is nevertheless necessary to clearly stipulate, in advance, the punishments associated with poor performance. In order for the motivational process to function properly, the individual must clearly perceive and understand the consequences associated with both good and poor performance. A more rational decision about work options can then be made.

Finally, as pointed out earlier, cost-effective nursing behaviors are often perceived as resulting in negative outcomes or punishments. This is obviously counterproductive. The example used to illustrate how this occurs involved a nursing unit that had been successful in reducing its supply budget. The consequences that followed included a permanent reduction in their budget for the following year and demands for additional cuts. In such circumstances, motivating staff nurses effectively is almost impossible. Nurse managers must be aware of this potential problem and take steps to correct it when it occurs.

In summary, Step 1 of the motivational process involves stipulating clearly what behaviors are expected of staff members, along with the consequences associated with different levels of performance. The purpose is to explicitly communicate performance expectations and performance–outcome contingencies. The effective accomplishment of this step is essential to the success of the entire process.

Step 2. Properly train and provide necessary support. After specifying performance expectations, nurse managers ensure that their staff has the training and support necessary to meet those expectations. As new, more cost-effective care practices are introduced, nurses must be adequately prepared and trained. This will typically involve continuing education programs designed to equip nurses with the requisite knowledge, skills, and abilities. Continuing education represents an immediate, short-term solution to the need for new skills. On a long-term basis, curriculum changes are needed in basic nursing preparation programs to ensure that graduates have the capacity to provide cost-effective patient care.

Once staff members are trained adequately, nurse managers must provide the support necessary to perform well. This assistance can take several forms, from funding, to personnel, to equipment, to moral/emotional support; in other words, the manager must do everything in her power to help her staff be successful.

By combining effective training with adequate support, the nurse manager hopes to convince staff members that trying hard can result in effective performance. Without this conviction, nurses will not be motivated to put forth a great deal of effort.

Step 3. Accurately measure performance behaviors. The old management adage mentioned earlier states that "if it isn't measured, it won't get done." This is certainly applicable to nursing. Motivating nurses to behave in more cost-effective ways requires that managers develop objective and accurate systems for measuring performance. Blaney, Hobson, and McHenry have demonstrated successfully that this can be done with cost-related practices in nursing.[27] Their approach and the complex issues involved are discussed in more detail in Chapter 6.

Without an acceptable system to accurately evaluate performance, motivating staff will be difficult, if not impossible. The nurse manager needs a valid way of identifying good and poor performers in order to equitably dispense rewards and punishments. In the absence of such a system, incentives cease to motivate behavior.

Step 4. Provide valued rewards/punishments contingent on performance. The fourth and final step in the expectancy theory-based motivation process involves actually dispensing rewards and punishments based on performance, as promised in Step 1. Good performers, those who meet or exceed behavioral expectations, should receive promised incentives. The consequences of failing to provide these rewards are disastrous. Likewise, failure to deliver punishments to poor performers can lead to major disciplinary and motivational problems.

The poor performer presents a special challenge to any supervisor. The key issue with such individuals is to discover the reason for the poor performance. Is it due to a lack of ability, effort, or a combination of the two? In most cases, lack of ability can be dealt with effectively through retraining and counseling. An employee might occasionally require a reassignment to a different or a lower level job. As long as the person is trying hard to succeed, most managers and organizations will work with them and find an appropriate position.

On the other hand, if poor performance is primarily a function of a lack of effort, an entirely different response from the manager is appropriate. Initially, counseling is recommended as a means of discovering why the person is not trying and attempting to correct the situation. If this fails, perhaps retraining or reassignment to a different job might help. In many cases, however, the supervisor has no choice but to begin using the progressive disciplinary process, which involves increasing the severity of punishment for each additional occurrence of unacceptable performance.

Nurse managers can no longer afford to tolerate staff members who refuse to improve the cost-effectiveness of their own performance and who oppose the supervisor's authority. Although such cases should occur only infrequently, they must be dealt with decisively. If the person refuses to cooperate and change, dismissal (with appropriate work-related documentation) is unavoidable.

Staff members must realize that the manager controls and dispenses valued rewards and punishments based on demonstrated performance. Those who cooperate and improve the cost-effectiveness of their performance will be rewarded, whereas those who refuse to cooperate will be punished, and will ultimately be discharged.

Successful staff motivation programs can thus be developed by following the four-step process outlined above. Without a doubt, this will require a great deal of effort and hard work on the part of the nurse manager. The payoff, however, is substantial. Staff members will firmly believe that (1) trying hard results in effective performance and (2) valued rewards are provided to successful performance. According to Vroom, when this occurs, staff nurses will be maximally motivated to provide high quality, cost-effective patient care.

SUMMARY AND CONCLUSIONS

1. Effectively meeting the challenges offered by the new demands for cost containment in health care will require that nurse managers be able to successfully motivate their staff.

2. Motivation can be defined as the set of psychological processes that energize a person's behavior, direct it toward attaining some goal, and sustain it over time. From the perspective of nurse managers, this definition translates into three important motivational questions: (a) what can be done to get nurses excited about improving the cost-effectiveness of patient care, (b) what can be done to encourage nurses to learn and use new cost-effective practices, and (c) what can be done to ensure that new cost-effective practices continue to be used?

3. Intrinsic motivation can be defined as motivation to engage in an activity for which there is no apparent reward except for the activity itself, whereas extrinsic motivation involves engaging in an activity for the material outcomes that it brings. Generally, people work better and harder when they are intrinsically motivated. Nurse managers should thus attempt to develop and foster intrinsic motivation among their staff with respect to the necessary behavioral changes associated with providing more cost-effective patient care.

4. The expectancy theory of work motivation has generated the most consistent research support of any comprehensive approach to human motivation. Within this theory, motivation to put forth a high level of effort on a particular task is a function of two major factors: (a) the person's subjective belief that trying hard will lead to successful performance, and (b) the person's perception of the successful performance will result in valued rewards.

5. Implementing expectancy theory in practice is relatively straightforward and involves the following four steps: (a) specifying and clarifying performance expectations and outcomes, (b) properly training staff members and providing necessary support, (c) accurately measuring performance behaviors, and (d) providing valued rewards/punishments contingent on performance.

6. Reward programs can be structured at any one of three levels — individual, group, and organization-wide. Each has its own advantages and disadvantages. An ideal approach involves providing rewards at all three levels in order to maximally motivate individual performance, encourage work group cooperation, and facilitate interdepartmental team work.

7. Incentives consist of two basic types—monetary and nonmonetary. Monetary incentive systems include the following: (a) piece rate, merit pay, merit bonus, and salary *vs* hourly wages at the individual level, (b) gain sharing at the group or departmental level, and (c) profit sharing and stock ownership at the organization-wide level. Major nonmonetary incentives include the following: recognition, advancement and promotion, participation in decision making, autonomy, task rotation and skill variety, task completion, feeling of belonging and usefulness, understanding and help with personal problems, professional development opportunities, and time banking.

8. Unfortunately, the current motivational climate in nursing, with respect to encouraging new cost-effective behaviors, is less than adequate. Many nurses associate cost-effectiveness directly with negative outcomes (*e.g.,* poor quality care, working harder, layoffs) or with the avoidance of negative outcomes (*e.g.,* I won't lose my job, the hospital won't go out of business). Incentives and rewards must be clearly linked to good performance in order to successfully motivate nurses to practice new behaviors. Some encouraging signs are available, suggesting that nurses recognize the need to provide valued outcomes to those who exhibit cost-effective behaviors.

9. A comprehensive action plan for nurse managers involves implementing the four-step expectancy theory process in order to motivate staff nurses. This includes (a) carefully specifying expected performance behaviors to include a quality component, (b) delineating the rewards (both monetary and nonmonetary) and punishments associated with different levels of performance, (c) providing necessary training and support, (d) accurately measuring performance behaviors, and (e) dispensing rewards and punishments based on staff performance.

Questions for Reflection and Discussion

1. What is the definition of motivation and how can it be translated into three important motivational questions or nurse managers? Discuss the relative difficulty of the energizing, directing, and sustaining components with respect to cost-effectiveness. Which of these do you feel possess the greatest challenge to nurse managers?

2. What is the difference between intrinsic and extrinsic motivation? Give an example of a situation in which you were motivated intrinsically to perform a particular task. Why is

it important for nurses to be motivated intrinsically? Finally, what can a nurse manager do to develop and foster intrinsic motivation in her staff?

3. Describe the two basic components in Vroom's expectancy theory and give a personal example to illustrate how the theory operates in practice.

4. Describe the four steps involved in applying expectancy theory in the work place. Give an example of how you would use it to motivate someone working for you.

5. Briefly discuss the three levels at which reward programs can be structured and present the major advantages and disadvantages of each. Which do you think would work most effectively in nursing? Give reasons for your answer.

6. Which of the different types of monetary incentive plans do you feel would be most useful in nursing? Give reasons for your answer.

7. In your opinion, what are the most important types of non-monetary incentives and how do they affect intrinsic motivation?

8. How would you evaluate the current motivational climate in nursing with respect to cost-effectiveness? Would you agree that many nurses perceive that punishment and the avoidance of punishment are major outcomes associated with cost-effectiveness programs? What positive outcomes do nurses associate with cost-effectiveness? How did these nursing perceptions and beliefs develop and what can be done to change them?

9. What specific advice would you give to a head nurse regarding how she should use expectancy theory in motivating staff members? How would you measure job performance and how would you reward good performers? How would you deal with chronically poor performers?

REFERENCES

1. Deci EL: Intrinsic Motivation. New York, Plenum, 1975
2. Hobson CJ, Meade ME, Soverly D: CE: Out-dated notions can't update nurses. Nurs Man 16:35–38, 1985
3. Baron RA: Behavior in Organizations, 2nd ed. Boston, Allyn & Bacan, 1986
4. Ivancevich JM, Matteson MT: Organizational Behavior and Management. Plano, TX, Business Publications, 1987
5. Miner JB: Theories of Organizational Behavior. Hindsdale, IL, The Dryden Press, 1980
6. Vroom VH: Work and Motivation. New York, Wiley, 1964

7. Steers RM, Porter LW: Motivation and Work Behavior, 4th ed. New York, McGraw–Hill, 1987
8. Peters TJ, Waterman RH Jr: In Search of Excellence. New York, Harper & Row, 1982
9. Arvey RD, Ivancevich JM: Punishment in organizations: A review, propositions, and research suggestions, Acad Man Rev 5:123–132, 1980
10. Hamner WC: Reinforcement theory and contingency management in organizational settings. In Tosi HL, Hamner WC (eds): Organizational Behavior and Management: A Contingency Approach. Chicago, St. Clair Press, 1974
11. Whyte WF: Skinnerich theory in organizations, Psychol Today 5(11):67–68, 96, 98, 100, 1982
12. Wiard H: Why manage behavior? A case for positive reinforcement. Hum Resource Man 11(2):15–20, 1972
13. Adams JS: Toward an understanding of inequity. J Abnorm and Soc Psychol 67:422–436, 1963
14. Mowday RT: Equity theory predictions of behavior in organizations. In Steers RM, Porter LW (eds): Motivation and Work Behavior, 4th ed. New York, McGraw–Hill, 1987
15. Lawler EE: Pay and Organizational Effectiveness: A Psychological View. New York, McGraw–Hill, 1971
16. Business Week: How A&P fattens profits by sharing them. December 22, 1986, p 44
17. Hackman JR, Oldham GR: Motivation through the design of work: Test of a theory. Organizational Behavior and Human Performance 16:250–279, 1976
18. Hackman JR, Oldham GR: Work redesign. Reading, MA, Addison–Wesley, 1980
19. Hobson CJ, Hobson RB, Hobson JJ: Why managers use criticism instead of praise. Supervisory Management 30(3):24–31, 1985
20. DRG's: How many staff cuts ahead? Nurs Life 4(6):20–25, 1984
21. Labor letter. Wall Street J July 31, 1984
22. Madsen NL, Harper RW: Improving the nursing climate for cost containment. J Nurs Admin 15(3):11–16, 1985
23. Schnee EJ, Robbins WA, Robbins CL: Profit-sharing plans in non-profit hospitals. Nurs Man Feb. 24–27, 1986
24. Curry JP, Wakefield DS, Price JL et al: Determinants of turnover among nursing department employees. Res Nurs Health 8:397–411, 1985
25. McCloskey J: Influence of rewards and incentives on staff nurse turnover rate. Nurs Res 23:239–247, 1974
26. Gordon GK: Motivating staff: A look at assumptions. J Nurs Admin XII(11):27–28, 1982
27. Blaney DR, Hobson CJ, McHenry J: Improving the cost-effectiveness of nursing practice in a hospital setting. J Contin Educ Nurs (in press)

6

Understanding Performance Appraisal and Designing Systems to Monitor and Measure Nursing Behaviors

PERFORMANCE APPRAISAL is a general concept that includes the various approaches to measuring and evaluating work performance. It is a complex topic and one of the most heavily researched in personnel psychology.[1,2] Several excellent books are available that provide comprehensive reviews of the literature along with excellent practical suggestions.[3-5]

Performance appraisal is typically an emotionally charged issue for all parties involved. Subordinates dread the evaluative component and supervisors often wish to avoid the seemingly inevitable conflict that frequently results. Compounding this situation are several factors (*e.g.,* information processing deficiencies, biases, and prejudices) that make it difficult, if not impossible, to make comprehensive, accurate appraisals. Nevertheless, it is possible to design, implement, and use effective systems to measure nursing performance.

It can be argued cogently that no issue is more important in the effort to improve the cost-effectiveness of nursing practice than performance appraisal. There is an old saying in management, "If it isn't measured, it won't get done."

This certainly applies to cost-effectiveness in nursing. Administrators and supervisors can implore nurses to improve the cost-effectiveness of their performance, but until a system is developed to effectively measure these new expectations, lasting behavioral improvements will be difficult. If administrators and supervisors are really serious about the cost-effectiveness issue, they will invest the time, effort, and money necessary to devise effective appraisal systems to accurately measure cost-related nursing behaviors. Only when this is accomplished will the importance and seriousness of cost-effectiveness be clearly communicated to all nurses. Furthermore, only when this is done will it be possible to identify and reward nurses who behave in a more cost-effective manner and retrain and discipline those who do not. Functional performance appraisal systems are, from this perspective, essential to the success of any effort to improve the cost-effectiveness of nursing practice.

The purpose of this chapter is to provide a basic introduction to the area of performance appraisal and an overview of the salient issues that should concern nursing administrators, supervisors, and employees. The specific topics addressed include (1) the purposes of performance appraisal, (2) legal issues, (3) performance appraisal as a communication process, (4) the rater as an information processor, (5) the characteristics of an appraisal system, (6) a comprehensive performance appraisal program known as the POLYCAP system, and (7) the performance appraisal review session.

It is hoped that an understanding and appreciation of these topics will help nurses develop appropriate performance appraisal systems to support and facilitate increased cost-effectiveness in nursing practice.

PURPOSES

A well-designed performance appraisal system should accomplish four major purposes: (1) communicate performance expectations, (2) motivate employees to perform well, (3) facilitate individual employee development, and (4) provide information for organizational decision making concerning personnel. In the first instance, appraisal systems offer a useful framework for communicating performance expectations to all employees. The appraisal system should ideally specify the major dimensions of job performance, their relative importance, and exactly what constitutes unacceptable, acceptable, and superior performance on each dimension.

Information in this format should be provided to every employee and should be thoroughly discussed with her supervisor. If this communication process is followed correctly, employees will have a clear notion of what is expected of them in terms of specific performance behaviors.

The second major purpose of performance appraisal is that of motivating employees. Once performance expectations have been clearly identified and communicated, the appraisal system should motivate compliance with these expectations by providing rewards and punishments, contingent on performance.

As pointed out in Chapter 5, people do respond to incentives in the work place. A properly designed appraisal system should clearly identify the available incentives and structure the linkages or contingencies between good performance $\rightarrow$ rewards and poor performance $\rightarrow$ punishments. Once established, if these contingencies are followed (*i.e.*, good performers are rewarded and poor performers are punished), the appraisal system will function as a powerful tool to motivate employee performance.

Appraisal systems should also be designed to meet a third major purpose, that of facilitating individual employee development. In this sense, the appraisal system should be structured to identify major strengths and weaknesses in each employee's job performance. In collaboration with the supervisor, an employee's strengths should be emphasized and capitalized on, whereas specific strategies should be formulated for improvement in weak areas. Thus, in this instance, the appraisal process serves as a vehicle for the growth and development of individual employees.

Unfortunately, the evaluative component of the appraisal process is too often overemphasized at the expense of the developmental aspect. Supervisors must guard against this phenomenon and recognize the value of performance appraisal in further developing employees.

Finally, the fourth purpose of appraisal systems is that of providing information for decisions concerning personnel. In most organizations, common personnel decisions are based mainly on appraisal results. Such decisions typically include promotion, selection for training, retention, firing, raises, and bonuses.

A well-designed performance appraisal system can provide

invaluable information for use in making rational decisions about human resource utilization. Ideally, good performers should be accurately identified so that they can be treated differently than poor performers; that is, given raises and bonuses, promoted, selected for special training, and retained. Comprehensive performance information of this type is only available from a sound appraisal system.

In practice, it is difficult to design, implement, and utilize a performance appraisal system in such a way that these four purposes are all met completely. Often some are emphasized at the exclusion of the others. These basic purposes, however, should guide the conceptualization and development of any appraisal system and serve as goals to strive for.

LEGAL ISSUES

In the general area of performance appraisal, it is important that nursing administrators, supervisors, and employees have a basic understanding of the legal issues involved. Given the inherently subjective nature of the appraisal process as discussed earlier, human biases often find their way into performance ratings, frequently at the expense of minority members. Thus, one finds that minority individuals tend to receive consistently lower evaluation scores than majority members. For instance, research shows that blacks often receive lower evaluations than whites, and women lower than men. This kind of systematic bias and discrimination results in significant frustration and suffering, as well as the inefficient use of human resources. In addition, legal challenges to such biased appraisal systems can lead to tremendous costs to the guilty organization. These potentially include legal fees, court costs, adverse publicity, back pay and promotions, and mandatory affirmative action programs.

The substantial importance of legal issues in performance appraisal make it imperative that nurses have a fundamental knowledge of the basic concepts involved. As one might expect, the legal issues surrounding performance appraisal can be complicated and involved. Several books are available for the interested reader that provide comprehensive, yet straightforward and understandable, coverage of the key issues and legislation. Two of the more useful ones are those by Arvey and Ledvinka.[6,7]

The purpose of this section is to offer a brief and simplified overview of the most salient legal issues.

Federal regulations exist covering the use of performance appraisals with minorities, the elderly, and the handicapped. The focus in this section is restricted to the more prevalent and widely researched use of appraisals with minorities. It should be noted that similar, though less extensive material exists pertaining to the elderly and handicapped. The two books mentioned previously provide an excellent overview of these areas.

Federal Legislation

Title VII of the Civil Rights Act of 1964 (as amended by the Equal Employment Opportunity Act of 1972) provides the general framework for evaluating the legality of performance appraisal systems with respect to minorities. More detailed and specific information can be found in the Uniform Guidelines on Employee Selection.[8] The current federal regulations pertain to minority groups, termed *protected classes,* which are defined in terms of race, color, religion, sex, and national origin. This legal protection applies to all major employment decisions, including selection, retention, promotion, training, and raises.

As mentioned earlier, performance appraisals often provide critical information for personnel decision making. In fact, most organizations base promotion retention, training, and raise decisions mainly on appraisal results. This fact has led to the interest and legal scrutiny of the performance appraisal process.

Adverse Impact

Federal regulations have been designed specifically to monitor the "adverse impact" present in major organizational employment decisions. Adverse impact is defined generally as a rate of selection for employment, retention, promotion, or raise, and so forth, which works to the disadvantage of protected class members.

More specifically, adverse impact is defined in terms of the "four fifths rule" provided in the 1978 Uniform Guidelines on Employee Selection.[8] This rule states that the rate of selection for a protected class must be at least 80% (four fifths) as large as the rate for the majority group, or adverse impact is present. An example to illustrate this concept is provided in Table 6-1.

Table 6-1.   Adverse Impact Examples

	Eligible for Promotion	Actually Promoted	Promotion Rate
Protected class	100	20	20%
Majority group	100	50	50%

Data presented in the table indicate that 100 protected class members (*e.g.,* blacks, Hispanics, women) and 100 majority group members (typically whites or white men) are eligible for a performance-based promotion. In the protected class group, only 20 are actually promoted, for a promotion rate of 20%. Of the 100 majority group members, 50 were actually promoted, resulting in a promotion rate of 50%.

In applying the four fifths rule, one would multiply this majority group promotion rate by 80% (four fifths) to arrive at the minimally acceptable rate for protected classes. Eighty percent of the majority promotion rate of 50% is 40% ($0.8 \times 0.5 = 0.4$). Thus, protected classes must be promoted at the rate of at least 40% or an adverse impact will result.

In the example in Table 6-1, the protected class rate of promotion is 20%, well below the minimum requirement of 40%. Consequently, adverse impact would be charged in such case.

At this point, the organization involved would be obligated to demonstrate that its appraisal system met or exceeded federal regulations. If unsuccessful, the use of the appraisal system and promotional process could be declared illegal and the organization punished with such measures as court ordered back pay and promotions and mandatory affirmative action programs.

On the other hand, if the organization can successfully demonstrate that the appraisal system and appraisal process comply with federal regulations, it can legally continue to use them. Finally, in those situations where no adverse impact is found, organizations are not required to defend their appraisal and promotional processes, because they are assumed to be legal.

A summary of this information is provided in Table 6-2, in which adverse impact, compliance with federal requirements, and the legality of performance appraisal and promotional sys-

Table 6-2. Relationship Between Adverse Impact, Meeting Federal Regulations, and the Legality of Performance Appraisal Systems and Promotion Processes

	Federal Regulations Met	*Federal Regulations Not Met*
Adverse impact present	Legal	Illegal
Adverse impact not present	Legal	Legal

tems are related. As indicated in Table 6-2, the absence of adverse impact (in terms of the four fifths rule) results in the determination that an appraisal system and promotional process are legal. Likewise, meeting federal regulations also results in a positive finding of legality. The only situation in which a performance appraisal system and promotional process are judged to be illegal is when *both* adverse impact occurs *and* federal regulations are not met.

Review of Court Cases

Federal regulations and guidelines in the area of performance appraisal are complex and often open to differing legal interpretations. Consequently, one must rely on the accumulated body of case law and court decisions to ascertain exactly what is legally required.

Fortunately, two excellent reviews of major court cases are available by Cascio and Bernardin and Feild and Holley.[9,10] The two reviews draw essentially the same conclusions and provide a list of characteristics required to successfully defend an appraisal system in court.

Among these characteristics are the following:

1. Appraisal systems should be based explicitly on thorough job analyses.
2. Appraisals should be structured in terms of specific job behaviors and not traits (*e.g.,* initiative or dependability).
3. Raters should be given specific training on how to correctly use the appraisal system.

4. Appraisal results should be personally reviewed with each subordinate.

5. Subordinates should be given the opportunity to formally appeal appraisal results.

Although these factors will not guarantee success, they have characterized appraisal systems that have been effectively defended in court.

One final point about these legal requirements needs to be made. They should not be viewed as arbitrary and capricious governmental edicts, but rather constitute sound personnel practices. A rational, research-based approach to performance appraisal should include every item mentioned above. The federal government is not asking organizations to do anything that they should not already be doing in their own self-interest.

Nursing administrators need to be aware of the basic requirements of sound performance appraisal and incorporate them into their own organizational systems. If this is accomplished successfully, the legal issues will be simultaneously dealt with. Given the staggering potential costs associated with the use of faulty appraisal systems (*e.g.*, legal fees, court costs, adverse publicity, back pay and promotions, and mandatory affirmative action programs) it is imperative that the fundamental legal issues be understood and explicitly addressed by all nurses.

PERFORMANCE APPRAISAL AS A COMMUNICATION PROCESS

A major purpose of appraisal systems is the clear communication of performance expectations. If appropriately constructed, the appraisal system should specify and clarify exactly what is expected of all employees. Unfortunately, this communication process is rarely accomplished in an effective manner and is often beset with major problems and obstacles. In reality, a common complaint among employees in a wide variety of organizations and positions is that they do not know clearly what is expected of them on the job. Confounding this situation is the fact that supervisors are often not aware of these problems and thus cannot take the necessary steps to correct them.

In this section, four major problems in the performance appraisal communication process are presented and illustrated. Suggested solutions will then be discussed for each problem.

Supervisor Self-Insight

The first problem concerns the supervisor's own lack of accurate and consistent self-insight as to exactly what her performance expectations are. Research has shown that supervisors are frequently unaware of the manner in which they calculate performance ratings, both in terms of the factors taken into consideration and their relative importance.[11]

Supervisors typically report that they utilize and integrate many separate aspects of a subordinate's performance in arriving at their overall evaluation and that these aspects or factors are nearly equal in importance. For instance, a supervisor might report that ten factors are important in a subordinate's overall evaluation and that all are roughly similar in relative importance. An example of a typical set of self-report percentage weights, along with actual weights used in making ratings (as determined by a statistical analysis) is provided in Table 6-3.

Although the typical self-report pattern consists of (1) many individual dimensions of performance and (2) nearly equal percentage weighting, most supervisors actually use and combine performance information in a radically different manner. In fact,

Table 6-3. Comparison of Supervisor Self-Report Percentage Weights with Actual Percentage Weights Used in Making Ratings

Performance Dimensions	Supervisor Self-report Percentage Weights	Actual Percentage Weights Used by Supervisor in Making Overall Ratings*
1	10%	20%
2	5%	0%
3	15%	35%
4	10%	5%
5	10%	5%
6	5%	0%
7	10%	5%
8	15%	25%
9	10%	5%
10	10%	0%

*Based on a statistical analysis of the supervisor's rating behavior. More specifically, multiple regression is typically used to predict overall ratings from scores on individual performance dimensions and assess the relative contribution or importance of dimension.

for most supervisors, statistical analysis of their rating behavior would reveal that 3 to 4 performance dimensions are heavily relied on in the rating process and account for 75% to 80% of the overall appraisal. This common pattern is illustrated in the third column in Table 6-3, where the three largest weighted dimensions total 80% of the overall evaluation.

As mentioned in an earlier section, human beings are inefficient information processors and cannot accurately integrate a great deal of data on many different dimensions. Supervisors tend consequently to rely on and utilize only a few major dimensions in making their ratings.

Unfortunately, there is tremendous potential for miscommunication with subordinates concerning performance expectations. Most supervisors honestly believe that they are using multiple, approximately equally weighted, dimensions in making their overall evaluations and generally communicate this fact to subordinates. In reality however, overall ratings are actually based on only some of these dimensions.

This can lead to serious communication problems and conflict between supervisors and subordinates. For example, imagine that subordinates are told that the dimensions and weights in column 2 of Table 6-3 will be used in appraising their overall performance, while in fact, the dimensions and weights in column 3 are actually used. It is no small wonder then that subordinates often feel like they do not know exactly what is expected of them. The root of the problem is often the supervisor's own lack of self-insight into how she combines and weighs information in making appraisals and the failure to communicate accurate expectations to subordinates.

The solution in this situation involves first an awareness and recognition of the problem by supervisors. Once aware of the basic nature of the human information processing system, steps can be taken to thoughtfully and carefully specify performance dimensions and weights that accurately reflect the major duties of the job and the intentions of the supervisor. After specifying dimensions and percentage weights, this information should be communicated clearly to all subordinates. In addition, the supervisor must commit to using the specified dimensions and weights in the actual computation of overall ratings.

Verbal Dimensional Weights

A second related problem centers around the semantic ambiguity associated with the verbal weights often used by supervisors in describing the relative importance of various job dimensions. Exact statistical weights are rarely used in this process. Instead, supervisors typically use verbal descriptors such as "Most Important," "Very Important," and "Important."

To illustrate the nature of this problem, refer to the information contained in Table 6-4. Assume that you have just started a new job and the supervisor is describing the five major job dimensions, indicating their relative importance with the verbal labels given in the middle column of Table 6-4.

How would you interpret these verbal weights in terms of specific percentages? In other words, what percentage weights are equivalent to "Most Important," "Very Important," and "Important" in your opinion? Write in your answers and remember that the total of all five weights must be 100%.

As you might expect, responses to this exercise vary greatly from person to person. For example, the verbal label "Most Important" has received percentage weights ranging from a low of 25% to a high of 80% — a difference of 55 percentage points. Thus, some subordinates might be spending 25% of their time working on that job dimension, while others are spending 80% — and all of them would believe that they were correctly following the supervisor's guidelines.

Table 6-4. Percentage Interpretation of Verbal Importance Weights

Performance Dimensions	Verbal Importance Weights From Supervisor	Specific Percentage Weight
1	Most important	_____
2	Very important	_____
3	Important	_____
4	Important	_____
5	Important	_____
		(Total must add up to 100%)

Who is actually correct? There is no way of knowing unless the supervisor specifies what percentage weight she had in mind. Assume for a moment that the supervisor felt that 80% was the appropriate weight. What reaction would this supervisor have to subordinates who are only spending 25% of their time working in this area?

The resultant problems should be obvious and the potential for unnecessary confusion and conflict is high. Unfortunately, the same verbal weight has different meanings for different people. Whereas the supervisor might feel that she has clearly clarified the relative importance of the various job dimensions, nothing could be further from the truth!

The solution, however, is obvious and simple. Do not use verbal weights. When describing the relative importance of job dimensions, carefully conceived percentage weights should be given to subordinates. Only in this manner can the semantic ambiguity and confusion be dealt with effectively.

Subordinate Lack of Insight

Given the first two problems (supervisor lack of self-insight and the ambiguity of verbal weights), it is not surprising to find that subordinates often have little clear insight into exactly what the supervisor expects of them, either in terms of specific performance dimensions or their relative importance. This communication problem can be illustrated dramatically by completing the exercise contained in the box, Subordinate Job Assessment Form, and the box, Supervisor Job Assessment Form. It requires both the supervisor and subordinate to *independently* list the major dimensions of the subordinate's job, along with the associated percentage weights indicating the relative performance of each dimension. Try this exercise with your own supervisor and also with your subordinates, if applicable.

In all likelihood, you will be astonished at the lack of agreement, both in terms of the performance dimensions listed and their relative percentage weights. Supervisors and subordinates view the same job from systematically different perspectives, thus differences in perception should be expected to occur naturally, unless steps are taken to correct the situation.

It can be forcefully argued that a lack of agreement between supervisor and subordinate regarding the basic requirements of

SUPERVISOR JOB ASSESSMENT FORM

Directions

List the major dimensions of performance for your *subordinate's job.* Jobs typically have from 5 to 7 major dimensions, but not more than 10. For each dimension listed, indicate its relative importance to the job by assigning a specific percentage weight. These dimensional weights must total 100%.

Major Dimension of Performance	*Percentage Weights Indicating Relative Importance*
1. _____	_____
2. _____	_____
3. _____	_____
4. _____	_____
5. _____	_____
6. _____	_____
7. _____	_____
8. _____	_____
9. _____	_____
10. _____	_____
	Sum = 100%

SUBORDINATE JOB ASSESSMENT FORM

Directions

List the major dimensions of performance for your *own job.* Jobs typically have from 5 to 7 major dimensions, but not more than 10. For each dimension listed, indicate its relative importance to the job by assigning a specific percentage weight. These dimensional weights must total 100%.

Major Dimension of Performance	*Percentage Weights Indicating Relative Importance*
1. _____	_____
2. _____	_____
3. _____	_____
4. _____	_____
5. _____	_____
6. _____	_____
7. _____	_____
8. _____	_____
9. _____	_____
10. _____	_____
	Sum = 100%

the job is highly dysfunctional. In order to perform well from the supervisor's perspective, subordinates must first know clearly what the supervisor's performance expectations are.

Thus, to correct the problem of poor subordinate insight, it is the supervisor's responsibility to clearly and accurately communicate specific performance expectations, in terms of major dimensions and their relative importance. Ideally, there should be perfect agreement on these two factors between supervisor and subordinate. The responsibility for the success of this communication process clearly rests with the supervisor.

Performance Standards

A fourth and final problem often plaguing the communication component of appraisal systems is the fact that supervisors and subordinates rarely exhibit agreement on performance standards. In other words, the specific behaviors associated with different levels of job performance are frequently defined differently by supervisors and subordinates. Again, an exercise should help to illustrate the disagreement and confusion that typically exists.

A scale of measurement for a single major dimension of performance is provided in Figure 6-1. The scale ranges from a low of 0 to a high of 100. The supervisor and subordinate should independently complete the exercise by first agreeing on the performance dimension(s) to be scaled. Then, each person should indicate exactly how performance is measured on that dimension by identifying the specific job behaviors associated with the 100%, 75%, 50%, 25%, and 0% levels.

Try this exercise with your supervisor for the major dimensions of job performance, and with your subordinates, if applicable. In the typical situation, there will be little agreement regarding the specific behaviors associated with the various performance levels.

Once more, the responsibility for ensuring that the accurate communication of performance expectations occurs rests with the supervisor. A frequently suggested approach is to allow subordinates to participate in the process of determining specific performance standards to be used in the appraisal system. This has the desirable effect of encouraging system acceptance and commitment. Written performance standards, once established, should be communicated explictly to all subordinates.

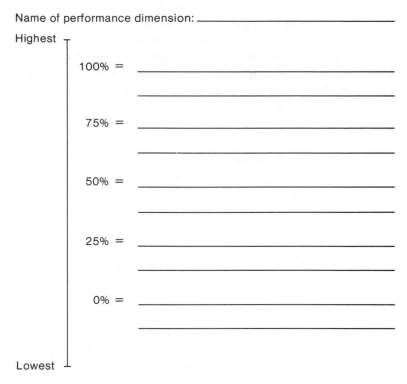

Name of performance dimension: _____

FIGURE 6-1. *Specific behavioral definitions of different levels of performance.*

A properly designed performance appraisal system should accurately, systematically, and comprehensively communicate performance expectations to subordinates. This requires that supervisors first fully understand their own performance expectations for subordinates and then successfully convey them to all employees. The process should ideally involve specifying the major dimensions of performance, their percentage relative importance, and the behavioral standards used to evaluate performance on each dimension. Only in this manner can the appraisal system meet its basic purpose of effectively communicating performance expectations.

RATER AS AN INFORMATION PROCESSOR

The task of completing performance appraisals places tremendous information processing demands on supervisors. They must first observe the performance of subordinates and through the processes of perception, attention, and memory form impressions of how well the individual is performing. These fragmented, incomplete impressions and observations are then combined and integrated in some manner to arrive at a single overall performance rating as required in most appraisal systems.

Unfortunately, research on human cognitive abilities and performance appraisal clearly indicates that raters are inefficient and biased information processors.[12,13] Data on subordinate performance are not comprehensively and systematically collected, but rather only selectively perceived, attended to, and processed. In addition, numerous "cognitive short-cuts" are used in processing performance information. Finally, a host of powerful biases and prejudices often contaminate ratings.

Landy and Farr, in their review of the performance rating literature, asserted that the information processing approach holds the key to future understanding of the basic underlying issues in performance appraisal.[14] The purpose of this section is to highlight the salient issues in this area and review some of the major information processing problems and biases that plague the appraisal process. An awareness of these problems is a necessary first step in developing effective solutions. Recognition of human inefficiencies can and should lead to the formulation of decision aids and performance evaluation formats that compensate for rater weaknesses.

Numerical Processing Inefficiency

Human beings have a distinctly limited capacity to process large amounts of numerical data, especially when asked to combine such information into a single summary number. This limitation causes major problems in appraisals when the rater attempts to combine a large volume of performance information into a single overall score at the end of the rating period. Very few, if any, people have the ability to do this accurately. Consequently, the use of simple mathematical decision aids can significantly improve the accuracy of the appraisal process.

An exercise designed to demonstrate the kinds of problems raters encounter is provided in Table 6-5. This exercise puts you in the role of a supervisor with five subordinates. It is the end of the year and time to give each of your subordinates an overall evaluation score from 1 to 100.

Table 6-5. Performance Rating Exercise

Performance Dimensions	Dimension Relative Importance	Profiles of Subordinate Scores From 1 to 100 on Each Separate Performance Dimension				
		Subordinate 1	Subordinate 2	Subordinate 3	Subordinate 4	Subordinate 5
1	15%	92	45	55	1	94
2	5%	34	62	35	19	49
3	5%	8	92	51	98	13
4	10%	47	5	65	78	99
5	5%	97	33	77	21	67
6	15%	15	21	89	67	95
7	5%	82	20	69	56	88
8	5%	50	75	74	13	65
9	25%	66	12	92	95	87
10	10%	23	25	86	49	79

Overall ratings (from 1 to 100):

Appendix to Table 6-5. Correct Answers, Scoring, Procedures, and Interpretation for the Rating Exercise

The "correct" ratings for each of the five subordinates are:

	Sub 1	Sub 2	Sub 3	Sub 4	Sub 5
	53	30	75	57	82

Percentage Weights		Dimension Scores		
0.15	X	92	=	13.8
0.05	X	34	=	1.7
0.05	X	8	=	0.4
0.10	X	47	=	4.7
0.05	X	97	=	4.85
0.15	X	15	=	2.25
0.05	X	80	=	4.0
0.05	X	50	=	2.5
0.25	X	66	=	16.5
0.10	X	23	=	2.3
		Total		53.0

These ratings were obtained by multiplying the percentage weights times the ten dimensional scores for each subordinate and then adding them up. For example, the overall rating of 53 for subordinate 1 was computed as shown at left. The sum of the scores in the third column represents the "correct" rating. In this case it is 53. Overall scores for the other four subordinates were computed in the same manner.

Now, for each of the five subordinates, compare your overall rating with the correct one and write down how far off you were; this is known as the *difference score.* The difference score is always positive and indicates how far apart two numbers are. If, for example, your overall rating for Subordinate 1 was 60, and the correct rating is 53, your difference score is 7 (60 − 53).

Next, add up the difference scores for the five subordinates. This is your total score and provides a rough index of your numerical information processing capacity. Scores have ranged from a low of 8 to a high of 123, with an average of 54. Total scores less than 25 are generally considered excellent, whereas those above 100 are considered poor. Scores between 25 and 100 are in the average range.

The key point to remember is that no one gets all of the ratings correct because human beings cannot efficiently or accurately process a great deal of numerical information. Decision aids are sorely needed. This case simply involves doing the necessary multiplication (percentage weights × dimensional scores) and addition. The message should be clear: do not trust something as important as performance evaluations to your fallible cognitive capacity to process numerical information.

The job involves ten major dimensions as indicated in the first column of Table 6-5. The second column of Table 6-5 contains the specific percentage weights associated with each dimension. For example, dimension 1 receives a weight of 15%, dimension 2 receives a 5%, and so on.

In preparation for making your final ratings, you have already evaluated each of the five subordinates on the ten separate performance dimensions. Thus, each subordinate has ten scores (from 1 to 100) on the individual dimensions. These scores are listed in the five columns under subordinate 1 to subordinate 5. For instance, subordinate 1 received a score of 92 (out of 100) on performance dimension 1, and subordinate 3 received a score of 74 on performance dimension 8.

Your task is to first review the scores on the ten performance dimensions for each individual subordinate. Then, using the percentage weights, combine that information into a single overall rating from 1 to 100. Write in your answers in the blanks provided at the bottom of Table 6-5.

In deciding on the overall ratings for each subordinate, do not use any calculations or computations. Do this task in your head, as is done by most supervisors. Also, do not spend more than 2 to 3 minutes on each person. When you have finished, turn to the Appendix at the end of Chapter 6 for the "correct" answers and scoring procedure.

You should find that your ratings differ (in some cases perhaps significantly) from the "correct" ratings computed using a simple mathematical decision rule given at the end of this chapter. This exercise should convince you that human beings are not efficient information processors and that they consequently need to develop decision aids to compensate for these limitations.

Supervisors have an obligation and responsibility to their subordinates to formulate overall performance ratings as accurately and efficiently as possible. In most cases, this necessitates the use of systematic decision aids, such as the formula used in computing "correct" answers in the rating exercise.

A final question should drive this point home. Knowing what you know now, would you like your supervisor to formulate your overall performance rating in her head, without the use of any decision aids?

Memory, Cognitive Categorization, and First Impressions

In a seminal article in 1981, Feldman summarized and integrated a great deal of research in the areas of cognitive psychology, information processing, and performance appraisal.[15] His major findings are intriguing and underscore the limitations and biases inherent in the appraisal process.

Feldman begins by pointing out that the typical annual appraisal is determined largely by the supervisor's memory of the subordinate's performance, not the actual performance itself. Over the course of the rating period, the supervisor observes instances of performance and encodes them for memory. Only events that have been properly encoded and stored will be recalled at appraisal time and influence the overall rating. From this perspective, human memory plays a critical role in the appraisal process and should, according to Feldman, be more systematically addressed.

He continues to summarize the existing literature on human memory and how it affects appraisal results. Interestingly, memory of subordinate performance is influenced strongly by the first impression made by the individual on the supervisor.

Research has shown that first impressions are made quickly (often under 5 minutes) and are based primarily on nonverbal cues, such as attire, grooming, facial expressions, posture.[16,17] Feldman argues that, based on first impressions, subordinates are quickly assigned to one of a limited number of mental categories used by the supervisor to classify people and subordinates.

The use of such cognitive categories enables the supervisor to more efficiently and quickly organize information about subordinates. Rather than considering and remembering each subordinate as a unique individual, they are represented as members of a well-defined category of subordinates. Every person in the category is assumed to possess the same salient characteristics.

To illustrate the categorization process, recall the portrayal of Archie Bunker by Carroll O'Connor in the television series *All in the Family*. How many cognitive categories for classifying people did Archie have and how quickly did this process occur?

As with most people, Archie had a relatively small number of categories into which most people could be quickly classified. For instance, the White-Anglo-Saxon-Protestant (WASP) category to which Archie belonged consisted of those people who were similar to him in terms of such things as ethnic heritage, sex, skin color, and political views. People who were different from Archie were generally categorized into less than positive groups. Over the years, these included such categories as blacks, Hispanics, Catholics, communists, hippies, and homosexuals. Archie quickly sized up an individual, put that individual into a category, and then treated him as if he had all of the characteristics of persons in that group. While obviously a caricature of the person categorization process, it is nevertheless a remarkably accurate representation of what typically occurs.

Feldman contends that initial subordinate categorization has important implications for a supervisor's memory of that person's performance. Several interesting and startling phenomena occur based on the initial categorization process. The interrelationships among these factors are summarized in Figure 6-2.

1. Supervisors show a tendency to selectively perceive and attend to information that confirms the initial categorization. Inconsistent information will tend not to be perceived or attended to. Thus, if an individual is categorized initially as a poor performer, supervisors will selectively perceive and pay attention to information that reinforces this categorization and they will ignore inconsistent data.

2. Over time, supervisors tend to demonstrate enhanced memory of behaviors and events consistent with the initial categorization and weakened recall (selective forgetting) of inconsistent information. Supervisors thus seem to better remember those events that confirm their initial categorization of a subordinate and quickly forget inconsistent data. One often observes this phenomenon in operation in work settings. For example, with a person initially categorized as a poor performer, instances of failure will be remembered very well by the supervisor and instances of success will be more quickly forgotten. Likewise, with good performers, supervisors tend to better remember successes more than failures.

3. Supervisors exhibit a tendency to actively search for information that confirms the initial categorization of a subordinate. People like to view themselves as accurate judges of others and will often go to great lengths to substantiate their initial opinions.

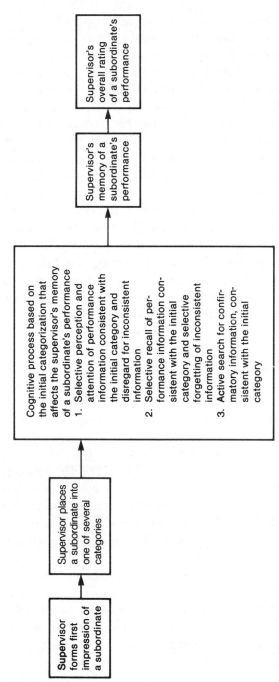

FIGURE 6-2. *The role of first impressions, initial categorization, cognitive processes, and memory as determinants of performance appraisal ratings.*

The aforementioned processes dramatically illustrate the selectivity, simplification, inefficiency, and bias ingrained in the appraisal process and the important role of memory and first impressions. Supervisors and subordinates should be aware of these phenomena and develop conscious strategies to deal effectively with them. For example, one excellent supervisory strategy to overcome the problem of selective memory involves maintaining a performance file or diary for each individual subordinate. This document should contain a chronologic listing of major instances of both poor and good performance. Such information can serve as an excellent record of a subordinate's performance and is invaluable in completing overall evaluations. Supervisors should not trust their memories, but they should rather rely on a systematic written record of specific performance behaviors.

From the subordinate's perspective, it is important to fully document all successes and ensure that the supervisor has a written copy of this information prior to formulating overall evaluations. This advice is especially relevant for someone who was categorized initially as a poor performer.

One final interesting point about the person categorization process is that supervisors and people in general tend to resist recategorization. Once a subordinate has been categorized, the supervisor is often reluctant to reclassify the individual, even in view of what appears to be overwhelming evidence to the contrary.

Everyone has probably seen this occur in the work setting at some point. For instance, if you "get off on the wrong foot" with the supervisor and are categorized as a trouble maker or poor performer, it is difficult, if not impossible, to change the supervisor's mind. Similarly, a subordinate who is categorized as a good worker will often be defended by the supervisor despite numerous examples of poor performance.

Of course, there are limits to this phenomenon and recategorization does occur. However, the point is, recategorization is done reluctantly. Consequently, the advice to subordinates is to try to make a good first impression on your employer and take advantage of being placed in a positive category.

Rating Errors

Extensive research in personnel psychology has documented the tendency of supervisors to commit a number of systematic information processing errors when making ratings.[3-5] Supervisors and subordinates should be aware of the major potential problems and they should develop strategies to deal effectively with them.

The three most salient rating errors are presented and discussed in this section. Although many other types of rating error have been identified, the following three errors are generally considered to be the most significant.

HALO ERROR

Perhaps the most prevalent of all rating errors, halo error results when a supervisor allows her evaluation of a subordinate on only one or a few specific performance dimensions to affect the overall evaluation. For instance, if a supervisor knows that a nurse has excellent clinical knowledge, this may lead to a positive overall rating, including high scores on all other major dimensions of performance. If this is the case, the halo is said to be *positive.* On the other hand, if a supervisor's overall evaluation of a subordinate is influenced by the knowledge of a nurse's poor performance on one or a few individual job dimensions, the halo is termed *negative.*

This phenomenon is one of many examples illustrating how supervisors simplify the appraisal process. Rather than taking the time or energy to assess every performance dimension individually, supervisors frequently assume that if a person is high on one or a few dimensions, she is probably also high on others and is thus a good performer overall. This type of rating error obviously ignores the complexity and heterogeneity of individual competencies.

CONTROL TENDENCY ERROR

This type of error involves unrealistically restricting overall subordinate performance ratings to the middle or central range of the measurement scale. Subordinates are all rated as approximately average, with no one receiving very positive or negative scores.

Again, this reflects a disinclination to more thoroughly conduct appraisals and realistically determine overall evaluations. Instead, it is easier to give everyone an average score so that no one is really happy or upset.

Control tendency error, however, penalizes good performers

with average ratings and rewards poor performers with the same ratings. This method is clearly dysfunctional from a motivational perspective.

LENIENCY/SEVERITY ERROR

This error involves a tendency on the part of the supervisor to give unrealistically high (leniency) or unrealistically low (severity) ratings to all subordinates. With the lenient supervisor, everyone receives good evaluations, thus incorrectly rewarding poor performers. The severe rater gives low evaluations to everyone, thus incorrectly penalizing good performers. Both varieties are obviously undesirable in terms of optimally motivating subordinates.

For those who completed the rating exercise in Table 6-5, it is possible to get a rough indication of your position on the leniency/severity dimension. Look again at your five overall ratings and compare them to the five correct ones. If four or five of your ratings were larger than the correct ratings, you exhibit a tendency to be a lenient rater. On the other hand, if four or five of your ratings were lower than the correct ones, you exhibit a severe rating tendency. Score patterns in between these two extremes suggest that you do not neatly fit into one of the two categories, but are instead less systematic in your inefficiency.

Efforts to train raters to control rating errors in performance appraisals have met with some limited success. It is possible to develop training programs that result in fewer rating errors. Interested readers should refer to the articles by Bernardin and Buckley and Smith for reviews of the rater training literature.[18,19] An awareness of these kinds of rating errors is a necessary first step in developing strategies to control and limit them.

Attribution Theory and Actor/Observer Bias

One final aspect of the human information processing system that has important implications for performance appraisal is the area involving attribution theory and the actor/observer bias. The concept of attribution has been formally developed by several researchers, including Heider, Jones and Davis, and Kelley.[20–23]

Attribution theory deals generally with the process by which people try to understand the causes of the behavior of others.

When evaluating another person's actions, there are many potentially valid causal explanations.

For instance, if a nurse reported that she recently received a grade A in a nursing course at the local university, several causal possibilities exist. Perhaps the nurse is smart, or worked hard, or received assistance from classmates, or was lucky, or the course material was simple, or the instructor was easy. The point is that many different explanations or attributions are possible.

Within attribution theory, causal explanations are generally grouped into two major categories: internal and external. *Internal attributions* refer to causes originating within the individual and typically include such factors as effort and ability. Continuing with the example above, if the grade of A is attributed to the nurse's ability to hard work, an internal attribution is made.

External attributions, on the other hand, refer to causes originating outside of the individual. For instance, when the grade A is attributed to help from classmates, luck, a simple course, or an easy instructor, the attribution made is an external one.

Research has shown that people tend to make certain kinds of attributions depending on the target person in question.[24] When making attributions concerning one's own behavior, people show a marked tendency to emphasize external factors and minimize internal ones. In contrast, when analyzing another person's behavior, people tend to make internal as opposed to external evaluations. This basic phenomenon is known as the *actor/observer bias.* People generally overemphasize the external causes of their own behavior and the internal causes of others' behavior.

The actor/observer bias has significant implications for the performance appraisal process, especially with regard to instances of poor subordinate performance. When an employee makes a mistake or does a poor job, what kind of attribution is typically made by the supervisor — internal or external? In most cases, supervisors automatically make an internal attribution, asserting that the cause was a lack of effort or ability or some combination of the two. External factors tend to be overlooked or minimized.

In contrast, what kind of self-attribution is typically made by the subordinate concerning her own poor performance — internal or external? People generally make external attributions and blame the poor performance on such factors as task difficulty, lack of support or resources, poor luck, lack of cooperation from other people, or outside interference and obstacles. The list of external attributions is endless. In this self-attributional process, the role of internal causes is minimized, because people rarely view themselves as the primary cause of a problem.

The contrasting attributions made by supervisors and subordinates are depicted in Figure 6-3. The opportunity for misunderstanding and conflict is obvious. Whereas the supervisor overemphasizes internal causes, the subordinate overemphasizes external ones. Typically, in most situations the true state of affairs lies somewhere in between these two extremes.

Supervisors should be aware of this nearly automatic tendency on their part to attribute subordinate performance failures to internal causes, while at the same time overlooking external ones. More careful consideration should be given to the potentially important external factors that often play a major role in determining success or failure.

Supervisors should also anticipate that subordinates will

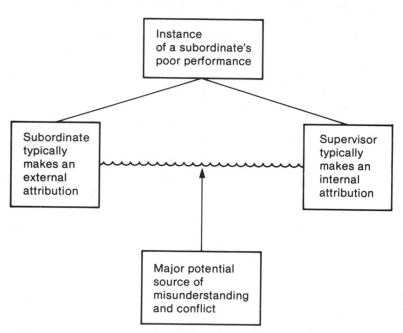

FIGURE 6-3. *Supervisor's and subordinate's differing attributions for a subordinate's poor performance.*

usually attribute their own performance failures to primarily external causes. This anticipation can help reduce the likelihood of misunderstanding and conflict with the subordinate.

Interestingly, the knowledge of this phenomenon can also work to the subordinate's advantage. When a mistake is made, what course of action would you recommend?

Knowing that the supervisor tends to make internal attributions and expects the opposite from the subordinate, an effective and disarming technique is to immediately accept personal responsibility, apologize, and not offer any excuses. Coupled with a sincere promise not to make the same mistake again, this tactic can serve to effectively defuse an otherwise explosive situation.

The typical supervisor is often caught completely off guard and is rendered speechless. Once an individual has genuinely acknowledged her own personal responsibility or guilt, apologized, and pledged not to make the mistake again, most supervisors will completely accept the apology and will work with the subordinate to help improve her performance. Certainly, the supervisor will find it difficult to continue to chastise or criticize the subordinate.

If you have never tried this strategy as a subordinate before, the next time you make a blunder, use this approach and observe what happens. The outcome with most supervisors is predictable and positive.

Practical applications of this basic psychological process can be found in many areas of human interaction. The combination of admitting guilt and apologizing tends to elicit an understanding and sympathetic response from most people. Numerous public figures and politicians have used this knowledge to their benefit. One notable exception is Richard M. Nixon. Had he followed this advice following Watergate, and had he admitted guilt and apologized, in all likelihood the American people would have forgiven him and he would have served out his full term in office.

CHARACTERISTICS OF EFFECTIVE PERFORMANCE APPRAISAL SYSTEMS

Many researchers and writers have studied and investigated the factors characterizing successful and effective performance appraisal systems. Cascio summarized and integrated this literature by presenting five fundamental requirements that should be met by any appraisal system.[25]

Relevance

This characteristic pertains to the relationship between a performance appraisal system and the actual requirements of the job. A relevant system should be based clearly on a thorough job analysis and should accurately reflect the various behaviors necessary for success.

Sensitivity

An effective appraisal system must be sensitive enough to distinguish between good and poor performers. The system should facilitate the process of identifying good performers for subsequent reward and poor performers for retraining or discipline. It is essential that the measuring capability of the appraisal system be accurate or sensitive enough to detect such differences in performance level.

Reliability

The third characteristic concerns the consistency with which appraisal evaluations are made. Ideally, multiple supervisors, working independently of one another, should arrive at basically the same overall rating for a particular employee. Similar evaluations would indicate a high degree of inter-rater reliability or consistency in the appraisal system. Reliability is a basic requirement for any measuring device, and the entire appraisal system is useless without it.

Acceptability

From a pragmatic perspective, the most important characteristic of an effective appraisal system is that it is accepted by the supervisors and subordinates who will be using it. A system that is not accepted will not be used properly and is thus largely ineffective. Supervisors and subordinates must view the appraisal system as reasonable and acceptable.

One excellent method to improve a system's acceptability is to involve all concerned parties in the planning and developmental stages. For instance, by allowing for active participation and input from supervisors and subordinates, the likelihood that the appraisal system will be accepted can be significantly increased.

Practicality

The fifth and final characteristic of an effective appraisal system is practicality (*i.e.*, the extent to which the system is easy for supervisors to understand and use). Difficult, excessively complex appraisal formats are essentially useless. Given the busy schedules and multiple demands made on supervisors, a performance appraisal system must be simple, straightforward, and easy to use.

Designers and users of performance appraisal systems would be well advised to keep these five requirements in mind. Although they will not guarantee success, failure to consider them adequately will make success difficult to achieve.

POLYCAP—A COMPREHENSIVE PERFORMANCE APPRAISAL SYSTEM

A systematic approach to performance appraisal known as *POLYCAP* is presented and discussed in this section. This program was first introduced by Hobson and Gibson.[26] It is based on extensive research in performance appraisal and has been successfully implemented and used by several different organizations from hospitals to grocery stores to public service agencies.

The system was designed to meet the basic requirements of sound performance appraisal and to comply with all governmental equal employment opportunity regulations. POLYCAP deals specifically with many of the problems confronting the appraisal process and offers raters a convenient, comprehensible, and useful format.

The POLYCAP system is designed as a participative approach to performance appraisal. Active involvement and input from supervisors and subordinates is encouraged at all phases in the program. Such participation will not only improve the quality of the overall system, but will also enhance program acceptance and commitment. Thus, in all cases, supervisors and subordinates are strongly recommended to actively participate in the development and implementation of the system.

POLYCAP is an acronym for "policy capturing"—a process

whereby a supervisor's rating policy is specifically defined or captured. A rating policy consists of the performance dimensions and associated weights used in making overall evaluations.

As mentioned in an earlier section, most supervisors have little clear insight into the precise nature of their rating policy. This causes major communication problems in the process of communicating performance expectations to subordinates.

The research on policy capturing and its applications to performance appraisal has attempted to carefully specify supervisor rating policies, to clearly communicate them to subordinates, and then to use the policy in making overall evaluations.[27]

The POLYCAP system consists of four basic steps, as listed in the box, Steps in the POLYCAP Performance Appraisal System.

Job Analysis

The first step involves an analysis of the major duties performed on the job. The objective is to identify and define the principal aspects or dimensions of the job. In order to be effective, the performance appraisal system must include all of the essential dimensions of performance and nothing more.

Important cost-related aspects of nursing performance must be included as job dimensions. The definitions of three significant cost-related dimensions of nursing performance, as reported in the study by Blaney and Hobson,[28] are provided in the box, Cost-Related Performance Dimension Definitions. These three performance dimensions were identified as significant determinants of the cost-effectiveness of nursing practice within the context of the particular hospital where the research was conducted.

As mentioned earlier, participation and input from supervisors and subordinates is strongly encouraged. In this first step, their contributions will ensure that the job analysis is complete,

---

STEPS IN THE POLYCAP PERFORMANCE APPRAISAL SYSTEM

1. Job analysis
2. Rating scale construction
3. Capturing or defining rater policies
4. Communication and use of rater policies

COST-RELATED PERFORMANCE DIMENSION DEFINITIONS

---

1. *Efficient use of supplies:* The extent to which the nurse is accurately aware of the cost of supplies used in providing patient care and efficiently uses these supplies in caring for patients.
2. *Optimal scheduling:* The extent to which the nurse schedules patient tests, procedures, and preparations to facilitate efficient processing and timely discharge.
3. *Goal setting and patient care plan:* The extent to which the nurse develops and actively uses a patient care plan consisting of explicit overall objectives to be met prior to discharge, along with specific daily goals that will result in timely discharge.

---

accurate, and not contaminated with irrelevant dimensions. The final result of this job analytic stage should be a set of non-overlapping performance dimensions that contain all of the major duties involved in the job.

Rating Scale Construction

Once the major dimensions of performance have been identified and defined through the job analysis, it is then necessary to develop a specific yardstick to measure performance on each dimension. Although several rating formats are available, it is essential that the scale be expressed in terms of specific job behaviors.[14,29] One of the most widely used and accepted behaviorally based scale formats is known as the behaviorally anchored scale (BARS).

First developed by Smith and Kendall,[30] BARS involves the participative development of rating scales for each dimension of performance using specific job behaviors (referred to as *anchors*) to represent the different levels of performance. For instance, actual job behaviors are sought which indicate good, average, and poor performance on a particular dimension.

The objective in this process is to reach an agreement between supervisors and subordinates regarding the behavioral definitions associated with the various levels of job performance. This agreement should be clearly established prior to the beginning of the rating period and can thus serve as a specific guide for subordinate performance efforts, explicitly describing expected behaviors on the major dimensions of the job.

In the Blaney and Hobson study,[28] BARS were developed for three important cost-related dimensions of nursing performance.

They are provided in Figures 6-4, 6-5, and 6-6. These scales indicate the specific behaviors that represent the 2, 5, and 8 performance levels on a 1 to 9 scale (lowest and highest). As such, they provide valuable direction to nurses in terms of cost-related performance expectations.

Capturing or Defining Rater Policies

Once the major performance dimensions have been identified and BARS developed for each, the next step involves explicitly defining the supervisor's rating policy. A rater's policy consists of the major dimensions of the job and the associated percentage weights.

Ideally, supervisors should involve subordinates in the process of determining dimensional weights to better ensure that they accurately reflect the relative importance of the individual dimensions in the overall job. Careful consideration should be given to this weighting process. Once decided on, the supervisors should commit to using the weights in the calculation of overall evaluation scores.

Communication and Use of Rater Policies

After carefully defining a supervisor's rating policy, the basic information should be communicated clearly to all subordinates in a written form. This material should include: (1) a list of the major dimensions of the job and their definitions, (2) the complete set of BARS for all performance dimensions, and (3) the percentage weights associated with each dimension.

Information in this format will provide subordinates with a clear and comprehensive set of behaviorally specific performance expectations, along with an explicit process and structure for conducting appraisals. However, in order for the POLYCAP system to function effectively, the supervisor must firmly commit to employing this framework in making overall ratings.

The use of the POLYCAP program in calculating overall evaluations is straightforward. First, the supervisor must assess a subordinate's performance on each of the major dimensions of the job, using the appropriate BARS (for computational ease, BARS can be constructed using a 1 to 100 scale, with behavioral anchors at the 100%, 75%, 50%, 25%, and 0% levels).

Once the dimensional BARS ratings have been made, they

(Text continues on p. 158)

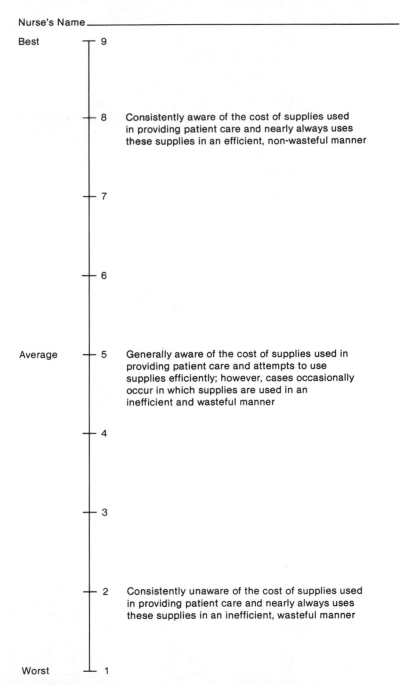

Nurse's Name

Best	9
	8 — Consistently aware of the cost of supplies used in providing patient care and nearly always uses these supplies in an efficient, non-wasteful manner
	7
	6
Average	5 — Generally aware of the cost of supplies used in providing patient care and attempts to use supplies efficiently; however, cases occasionally occur in which supplies are used in an inefficient and wasteful manner
	4
	3
	2 — Consistently unaware of the cost of supplies used in providing patient care and nearly always uses these supplies in an inefficient, wasteful manner
Worst	1

FIGURE 6-4. *Behaviorally anchored rating scale performance dimension: efficient use of supplies.*

Nurse's Name _____

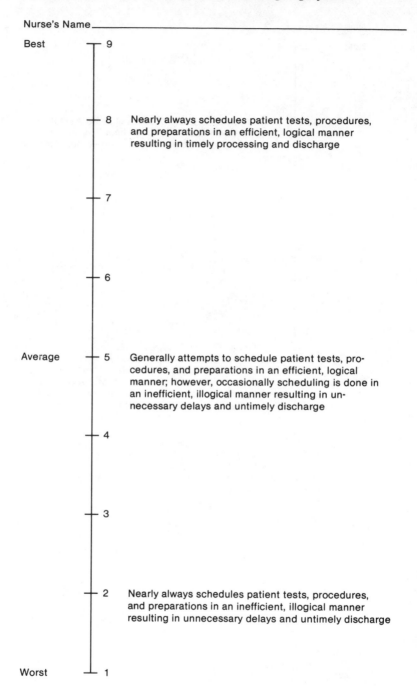

FIGURE 6-5. *Behaviorally anchored rating scale performance dimension: optimal scheduling.*

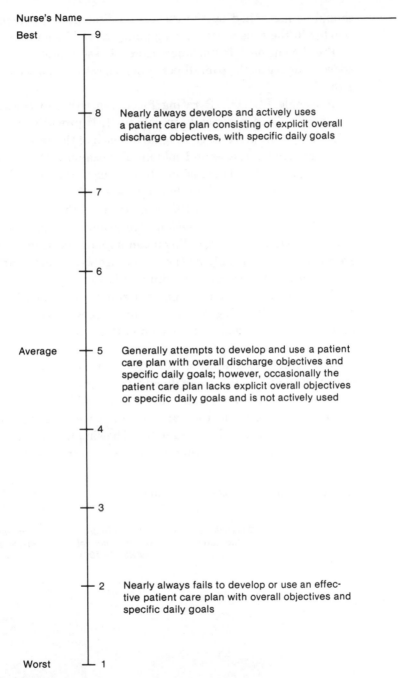

Nurse's Name _____

Best ⎯ 9

8 Nearly always develops and actively uses
a patient care plan consisting of explicit overall
discharge objectives, with specific daily goals

7

6

Average 5 Generally attempts to develop and use a patient
care plan with overall discharge objectives and
specific daily goals; however, occasionally the
patient care plan lacks explicit overall objectives
or specific daily goals and is not actively used

4

3

2 Nearly always fails to develop or use an effective patient care plan with overall objectives and
specific daily goals

Worst 1

FIGURE 6-6. *Behaviorally anchored rating scale performance dimension: goal setting and patient care plan.*

should be multiplied by the associated dimensional percentage weights in the supervisor's rating policy to yield what is known as the dimensional importance score. These scores should be added to arrive at the overall performance rating on a scale from 1 to 100.

A sample POLYCAP rating form, consisting of seven job dimensions listed generically in column 1, is provided in Table 6-6. The specific percentage weights for each of the seven dimensions are listed in the second column. For example, Dimension 1 has a weight of 30%, Dimension 2 has a weight of 20%, and so on through Dimension 7, which has a weight of 5%.

BARS ratings (on a 1 to 100 scale) made by the supervisor on each of the seven job dimensions are given in column 3. The fourth column contains the dimension importance scores, which are computed by multiplying the percentage weight for a particular dimension by the corresponding BARS score.

Thus, for Dimension 1, the importance score of 22.5 was obtained by multiplying 30% (the percentage weight) by 75 (the BARS score). The remaining six importance scores were calculated in a similar manner.

The overall evaluation scores (from 1 to 100) are then obtained by adding up the seven dimensional importance scores. In this case, the subordinate's overall rating would be 84.2.

Within this system, the same set of percentage weights is used consistently for all subordinates. The simple multiplication and addition preclude the mental processing errors often made

---

Table 6-6. Sample POLYCAP Rating Form

Performance Dimensions	Dimensional Percentage Weights	Rating Score on Dimensional BARS (1–100)	Dimensional Importance Scores
1	30%	75	22.5
2	20%	86	17.2
3	15%	95	14.25
4	15%	83	12.45
5	10%	98	9.8
6	5%	70	3.5
7	5%	90	4.5
			84.2
			Overall rating (1–100)

by supervisors in combining performance information into an overall score.

The overall POLYCAP system has several important strengths, including the following:

1. Solid research foundation
2. Emphasis on specific job behaviors
3. Compliance with all legal regulations
4. Specific measures to facilitate the clear communication of performance expectations
5. Special decision aids to overcome human information processing weaknesses

The system also offers several advantages to both supervisors and subordinates. From the supervisor's perspective the salient advantages include the following:

1. Clear, simple procedure for making overall ratings
2. Significant decrease in information processing demands
3. Increase in rating objectivity, consistency, and accuracy
4. Reduction in the likelihood of misunderstanding and conflict with subordinates

From the subordinate's perspective the major advantages are as follows:

1. Opportunity to participate in the development of performance expectations
2. Clarification of performance expectations in terms of specific job dimensions, percentage weights, and behavioral standards
3. Provision of a structured procedure for the computation of overall evaluations
4. Increase in rating objectivity, consistency, and accuracy
5. Reduction in subjectivity, bias, and prejudice in overall ratings

The POLYCAP program requires a substantial investment of time and energy to be correctly developed and implemented. However, it can be convincingly asserted that the benefits to both supervisors and subordinates, as well as the organization as a whole, are well worth the investment involved.

With respect to the issue of cost-effectiveness in nursing, the POLYCAP system offers an excellent opportunity to include critical cost-related behaviors within the context of a comprehensive performance appraisal format. Cost relevant dimensions of nursing practice must be clearly identified, defined, and included in the appraisal system. This is a necessary prerequisite for real progress and success in improving the cost-effectiveness of nursing practice.

PERFORMANCE APPRAISAL REVIEW SESSION

Most organizations require that formal performance appraisal results be communicated by the supervisor to the individual employee in a face-to-face meeting. This appraisal review session is often approached by both supervisors and subordinates with a great deal of reluctance and apprehension. The evaluative, critical component of the review session is typically resented by subordinates and supervisors find the resultant resistance and conflict to be distasteful.

In approaching the appraisal review session, it is important to keep in mind the four major purposes of appraisals mentioned earlier: (1) the communication of performance expectations, (2) the motivation of employees to perform well, (3) the personal development of individual employees, and (4) the provision of information for organizational personnel decision making. Performance review sessions offer an excellent opportunity to effectively address the first three purposes and these sessions should be structured and conducted with these purposes in mind.

A list of suggestions follows, which will increase the likelihood that the appraisal interview will accomplish its objectives and will be viewed as a positive, helpful, and constructive event both by supervisor and by the subordinate.

1. First, it must be emphasized that face-to-face performance feedback should not occur only at the annual review session. In order to optimally motivate and facilitate high levels of performance and goal attainment, periodic, informal performance feedback should be provided to all employees on a regular basis. Positive feedback should be given when subordinates are performing well. Corrective feedback is necessary when poor performance occurs. Frequent feedback is the best means of preventing unpleasant surprises in the review session.

2. In anticipation of the annual review session and the require-

ment for behaviorally based performance ratings, supervisors should maintain a diary or file for each subordinate, containing documented instances of especially good or poor performance. This material is invaluable in demonstrating to subordinates the rationale for a particular rating.

3. Prior to actually beginning work on a subordinate's overall evaluation, the supervisor should request a written self-evaluation from the individual. The subordinate should be instructed to review her own performance on the major dimensions of the job, highlighting significant accomplishments and strengths while also listing areas for further development. The self-evaluation can, if done properly, provide useful information and examples to the supervisor in completing the overall evaluation.

4. After receiving the subordinate's self-evaluation, the supervisor should formulate her written appraisal of the person's overall performance by documenting specific strengths and weaknesses and by arriving at a single overall rating. This written report should be provided to the subordinate prior to the actual review session, along with a statement that the report is a first draft and is subject to revision after the session. This allows the person to arrive at the meeting well prepared to discuss specific issues and concerns and ensures that there will be no major surprises.

5. At the beginning of the review session itself, the supervisor should make the subordinate feel as comfortable and relaxed as possible. The session should be conducted ideally in a quiet, private setting in an informal manner.

6. The supervisor should begin the session by highlighting the subordinate's major strengths and significant contributions. In addition, the supervisor should express her personal appreciation for these efforts and inform the individual of any recommended merit salary increases, bonuses, or promotions. It should also be emphasized that continued good performance will be rewarded to the best of the supervisor's ability.

7. Next, problem areas or weaknesses should be specifically discussed in behavioral terms, without resorting to personality issues. For example, rather than saying, "I don't like your attitude," it would be more appropriate to say, "Your consistent lack of punctuality for unit meetings is unacceptable." In all cases, actual job behaviors should be used to define and clarify areas of poor performance. It is especially critical during this stage in the appraisal interview to allow the subordinate to explain her perspective on these issues while the supervisor listens actively and attentively.

8. After discussing problem areas, it is imperative to jointly formulate and agree on concrete developmental or corrective strategies. A specific solution should be identified for each problem area. This joint problem solving orientation and approach will convey to the subordinate that the supervisor is concerned with helping her improve her performance.

9. The outcomes associated with continued poor performance and lack of improvement should be unambiguously communicated to the individual. Effective supervisors cannot and should not tolerate chronic poor performance and lack of corrective effort. Subordinates need to clearly understand what the associated consequences are.

10. The supervisor should ask how she could help the subordinate improve her job performance and then genuinely listen to the response. It goes without saying that supervisors look good when their subordinates do well. Consequently, it is in the supervisor's best interests to provide whatever support and assistance is necessary to help her subordinates be successful and improve performance behaviors.

11. Last, the supervisor should end the session by summarizing what has been said and by committing to a final revision of the written evaluation in a timely manner, taking into consideration what has been discussed. When completed, a copy of this final report should be provided to the subordinate, along with the opportunity to rebut it in writing.

If approached with these general guidelines in mind, the performance appraisal review session can be a positive and reinforcing process for both the supervisor and the subordinate. Ultimately, the success of the entire appraisal system depends on the supervisor's commitment to the rewards and sanctions promised in the review session. People do respond to incentives and behave according to their perceptions of available rewards and punishments. Consequently, it is essential that the supervisor follow through and deliver promised rewards to good performers and corrective or punitive measures to chronically poor performers.

SUMMARY AND CONCLUSIONS

A sound performance appraisal system is an essential ingredient in a comprehensive program to improve the cost-effectiveness of nursing practice. The old saying, "If it isn't measured, it won't get done," is certainly true today in nursing. If administrators and supervisors are serious about cost-effectiveness, they must invest the time, effort, and money necessary to incorporate cost-related job dimensions into a functional appraisal system.

A performance appraisal system should be designed to accomplish four major purposes: (1) the communication of performance expectations, (2) the motivation of employees to perform well, (3) the personal development of individual employees, and (4) the provision of information for organizational personnel decision making.

The characteristics necessary for an effective performance appraisal system include relevance, sensitivity, reliability, acceptability, and practicality.

Performance appraisal systems must meet various governmental equal employment opportunity regulations. All decisions based on appraisal results (*e.g.*, promotions, demotions, firing, training, raises, and bonuses) should be scrutinized for evidence of an adverse impact on members of protected classes. Where adverse impact is demonstrated (using the "four fifths rule), continued legal use of the appraisal system is contingent on proof that the system complies with governmental regulations. Reviews of recent court cases indicate that appraisal systems that have been defended successfully have had the following characteristics: (a) the appraisal system is based on thorough job analyses, (b) appraisals are structured in terms of specific job behaviors, (c) supervisors are trained in how to use the system, (d) appraisal results are personally reviewed with each employee, and (e) subordinates are given the opportunity to formally appeal appraisal results.

In terms of accurately communicating performance expectations, the appraisal process suffers from several major obstacles. Among the most important obstacles are the following:

(a) the supervisor's lack of self-insight into what performance dimensions and relative weights are used in making overall appraisals, (b) the semantic ambiguity and confusion surrounding the use of verbal weights to describe the relative importance of individual performance dimensions, (c) the subordinate's lack of insight into what performance dimensions and relative weights are used by the supervisor in making evaluations, and (d) the lack of agreement between supervisor and subordinate as to specific behavioral performance standards for the job.

The human information processing system affects the performance appraisal process in several significant ways:

a. Supervisors are generally inefficient at combining a great deal of performance data into a single overall rating.

b. A subordinate's overall evaluation is strongly influenced by the first impression made on the supervisor, the initial cognitive category the subordinate was placed in, and the supervisor's memory of subordinate performance over the rating period.

c. Supervisors tend to make several systematic rating errors; among the most prevalent are halo, central tendency, and leniency/severity.

d. Supervisors and subordinates systematically ascribe different attributions to the causes of subordinate performance. Known as the actor/observer bias, this phenomenon is often the cause of significant misunderstanding and conflict, especially when associated with instances of poor performance by the subordinate.

The POLYCAP system represents a comprehensive program to improve performance appraisal consisting of four steps: (a) a thorough job analysis, resulting in the identification and definition of major performance dimension, (b) the construction of BARS for all performance dimensions, (c) the description of supervisor rating policies in terms of job dimensions and percentage relative weights, and (d) the communication and use of supervisor rating policies in making overall evaluations. The program results in the unambiguous communication of behavioral performance expectations and simplified computation of overall ratings, as well as numerous specific benefits for supervisors and subordinates.

Both supervisors and subordinates often dread the performance appraisal review session. However, by following some simple guidelines, the review can be a positive event, serving to communicate and clarify performance expectations, motivate improvement, and develop subordinate job skills.

Questions for Reflection and Discussion

1. How important do you think performance appraisal is in promoting increased cost-effectiveness in nursing practice?

2. Do you agree with the old saying in management that, "If it isn't measured, it won't get done"? Can you give any examples to illustrate this?

3. In practice, how often do organizational performance ap-

praisal systems meet the four basic purposes presented in the chapter? What are the most common shortcomings and what can be done to correct them?

4. How can an organization determine if its performance appraisal system results in adverse impact in terms of the "four fifths rule" and is legal to use?

5. What characteristics should a performance appraisal system have in order to withstand a legal challenge and are these characteristics any different from those that a sound appraisal system should have in the first place?

6. How close is the agreement between you and your subordinates (or you and your supervisor) on: (a) the major dimensions of their job performance (or your job performance), (b) the percentage weights associated with these dimensions, and (c) the behavioral definitions of specific levels of performance on each dimension? Why do differences typically occur and what can be done to correct this problem?

7. How efficient are most supervisors in processing and integrating performance appraisal information? What decision aids would you recommend to help deal with this limited information processing capacity.

8. Why are first impressions, cognitive categorization, and memory so important in the performance appraisal process and how are they related? How does the initial cognitive category that a subordinate is placed in influence the supervisor's memory of that person's performance? Can you give any personal examples to illustrate these phenomena?

9. What are the major kinds of rating errors that supervisors make and how widespread and serious do you feel these problems are? Can you illustrate them with any personal examples? Also, how would you recommend that supervisors deal with these rating errors?

10. Do you believe that the actor/observer attributional bias is a major source of misunderstanding and conflict between supervisors and subordinates? Can you illustrate any of these problems with personal examples? What advice would you give to both supervisors and subordinates in terms of how to interact more effectively with each other, especially following instances of poor performance by the subordinate?

11. What is your assessment of the POLYCAP performance appraisal system? What are its strengths and weaknesses, and do you think it would work well in most nursing units? Would you like to use the POLYCAP system as a supervisor or as a subordinate?

12. In your opinion, why is the performance appraisal review

session so often a difficult experience for both supervisors and subordinates? How would you structure and conduct the review session to deal with these problems?

REFERENCES

1. Hakel MD: Personnel selection and placement. Ann Rev Psychol 37:351–380, 1986
2. Zedeck S, Cascio WF: Psychological issues in personnel decisions. Ann Rev Psychol 35:461–518, 1984
3. Bernardin HJ, Beatty RW: Performance Appraisal: Assessing Human Behavior at Work. Boston, Kent, 1984
4. Carrol SJ, Schneier CE: Performance Appraisal and Review Systems. Glenview, IL, Scott, Foresman, 1982
5. Landy F, Zedeck S, Cleveland J: Performance Measurement and Theory. Hillsdale, NY, Erlbaum, 1983
6. Arvey RD: Fairness in Selecting Employees. Reading, MA, Addison Wesley, 1979.
7. Ledvinka J: Federal Regulation of Personnel and Human Resource Management. Boston, Kent Publishing, 1982
8. Uniform guidelines on employee selection procedures. Federal Register 43:38290–38315, 1978
9. Cascio WF, Bernardin HJ: Implications of performance appraisal litigation for personnel decisions. Personnel Psychol 34:211–226, 1981
10. Feild HS, Holley WH: The relationship of performance appraisal system characteristics to verdicts in selected employment discrimination cases. Acad Man J 25:392–406, 1982
11. Hobson CJ, Mendel RM, Gibson FW: Clarifying performance appraisal criteria. Organizational Behav Hum Perform 28:164–188, 1981
12. Ilgen DR, Feldman JM: Performance appraisal: A process focus. Res Organiz Behav 5:141–197, 1983
13. Wesley KN, Klimoski R: Performance appraisal: An update. In Rowland KM, Ferris GD (eds): Research in Personnel and Human Resources, 2. Greenwich, CT, JAI Press, 1984
14. Landy FJ, Farr JL: Performance rating. Psychol Bull 87:72–107, 1980
15. Feldman JM: Beyond attribution theory: Cognitive processes in performance appraisal. J Appl Psychol 66:127–148, 1981
16. Arvey RD, Campion JE: The employment interview: A summary and review of recent research. Personnel Psychol 35:281–322, 1982
17. Knapp ML: Nonverbal Communication in Human Interaction, 2nd ed. New York, Holt, Rinehart, and Winston, 1978
18. Bernardin HJ, Buckley MR: A consideration of strategies in rater training. Acad Man Rev 6:205–212, 1981
19. Smith DE: Training programs for performance appraisal: A review. Acad Man Rev 11:22–40, 1986
20. Heider F: The Psychology of Interpersonal Relations. New York, John Wiley & Sons, 1958
21. Jones EE, Davis KE: From acts to dispositions: The attribution process in person perception. In Berkowitz L (ed): Advances in

Experimental Social Psychology, Vol 2. New York, Academic Press, 1965

22. Kelley HH: Attribution theory in social psychology. In Levine D (ed): Nebraska Symposium of Motivation. Lincoln, NE, University of Nebraska Press, 1967

23. Kelley HH: Attribution in Social Interaction. New York, General Learning Press, 1971

24. Jones EE, Nisbett RE: The Actor and Observer: Perceptions of the Cause of Behaviors. New York, General Learning Press, 1971

25. Cascio WF: Scientific, legal, and operational imperatives of workable performance appraisal systems. Public Personnel Man 11:367–375, 1982

26. Hobson CJ, Gibson FW: Capturing supervisor rating policies: A way to improve performance appraisal effectiveness. Personnel Admin 29(3):59–68, 1984

27. Hobson CJ, Gibson FW: Policy capturing as an approach to understanding and improving performance appraisal: A review of the literature. Acad Man Rev 8:640–649, 1983

28. Blaney DR, Hobson CJ: Development and psychometric analysis of a scale to measure attitude toward cost effectiveness in nursing. In Waltz CF, Strickland OL (eds): Measurement of Nursing Outcomes. New York, Springer (in press)

29. Schneider B, Schmitt N: Staffing Organizations, 2nd ed. Glenview, IL, Scott, Foresman, 1986

30. Smith PC, Kendall LM: Retranslation of expectations: An approach to the construction of unambiguous anchors for rating scales. J Appl Psychol 47:149–155, 1963

· PART TWO
Ability Factors
Necessary for Success

7

Basic Concepts in Financial Management and Budgeting

JOSEPH SCODRO

THE REVOLUTION occurring in the health care industry has focused increasing attention on the need for competent financial management and budgeting. Heightened competition, decreasing income, and rising expenses have combined to present hospitals in the United States with significant challenges. Health care institutions are responding by hiring financial experts, upgrading the skills of current managers, and introducing sophisticated new financial management and budgeting systems.

The ultimate success of these efforts to improve financial operations and cost-effectiveness hinges on the involvement and cooperation of nursing. The reason is that providing patient care remains the primary function of most hospitals and nurses play a predominant role in this process. Nursing must consequently be an active player in the drive for financial improvement.

In the past, hospital administrators often believed that nurses did not have the skills, inclination, or need to be involved in the financial operation of the institution. This belief was reinforced by the general lack of relevant course work at the undergraduate or graduate level in nursing and the unavailability of appropriate continuing education to provide needed skills.

Fortunately, this situation is changing dramatically. Nurses are demanding and obtaining a significant role in hospital financial operations. Administrators with insight have recognized that nurses are the real experts in improving the cost-effectiveness of patient care and their involvement is essential for success. Furthermore, nursing is finally being recognized as an important revenue-generating activity within the hospital.

In order for nursing to fully capitalize on this opportunity to influence the financial operation of the hospital, all nurses (including both staff and managers) must have a fundamental knowledge of the basic concepts and principles involved. Nurses must have an understanding of business. They must understand the financial operation of the hospital and the interrelationships among departments. But perhaps most important, they must be able to document the financial impact and importance of nursing care and take systematic steps to make improvements.

The basic purpose of this chapter is to introduce nurses to the key concepts and principles of financial management and budgeting, and how they apply in the health care environment. The focus is on understanding the reasons why financial management and budgeting are necessary and so important to the success of the institution in general and to nursing in particular. Only the most important concepts and principles are discussed. (For a more complete and comprehensive coverage of financial management and budgeting, see the references for Hoffman or Strasen.[1,2])

People in professions outside of accounting and finance typically approach these two subjects with a great deal of apprehension. This is also generally true of nurses. The specialized terminology and involved calculations frequently confuse and bewilder even the most serious student.

However, the fundamental concepts underlying financial management and budgeting are really simple and straightforward. Most people are implicitly aware of these concepts and use them in managing their own personal finances. Thus, we have found that an effective way to introduce and demystify the topics of financial management and budgeting is to use family finances as an example.

This approach has been applied successfully in numerous introductory accounting classes, as well as continuing education seminars for staff nurses and managers. Use of the family situation allows for the introduction of key concepts within a familiar nonthreatening context. These concepts can then be employed in understanding the operation of the hospital as a whole and individual nursing units.

FINANCIAL MANAGEMENT AND BUDGETING— A FAMILY EXAMPLE

All families engage in some type of financial management and budgeting, whether formally or informally. The process may be structured and systematic, or haphazard. The basic need for financial management and budgeting, however, is compelling. No family has an unlimited income or resources and there are many necessities of life and countless ways to spend money. Consequently, there must be some method of allocating resources to meet the needs of a family.

There are three basic relationships between a family's income and their expenses. First, if the total income exceeds the total expenses (a family earns $2,500 per month and expenses total $2,000), the family has a surplus. This enviable situation allows the family the option of spending the additional money or saving it.

On the other hand, if total income is less than total expenses, the family will incur debt in order to provide for basic needs. Nearly everyone has encountered a situation like this at some point in his life and it is normal. If, however, the losses are large or experienced for an extended time, the consequences can be serious, including: (1) an inability to pay bills at the correct time, (2) a poor credit rating, (3) repossession of items purchased on credit, (4) foreclosure on loans, and (5) eventual bankruptcy.

The third basic relationship between income and expenses occurs when they are equal (*i.e.,* no surplus or loss is experienced). The family would clearly prefer the situation in which income exceeds expenses. Proper financial management and budgeting can increase the likelihood that this can be achieved.

In the specific example in this section, a family of four (mother, father, and two teenaged children) has a combined monthly income of $1,500, with both parents working. As with most families, the process of financial management and budgeting had been accomplished in an informal and unsystematic manner. Assume, however, that the following three events have occurred that have changed their present financial requirements: (1) the family was notified that their rent would be increased by $50 per month, (2) the husband's work week was decreased from 5 days to 4, with a reduction in monthly pay of $100, and (3) the need for a second car within the next year became inevitable.

Faced with these circumstances, the family responded in the following manner. The parents called a meeting to discuss the problems, overall family objectives, and potential solutions. Each family member was required to participate and to offer his opinion. The rent increase and salary decrease were obviously inevitable and everyone agreed that a second car was desperately needed. A downpayment of $600 was required for this purpose.

Three general strategies were available to deal with these events. First, the family could attempt to increase its income. For example, the parents could seek better paying jobs or could take second, part-time jobs, or the teenagers could seek employment. The second approach involved reducing expenses, and the third approach involved trying simultaneously both to increase income and to decrease expenses.

For purposes of this example, the family unanimously decided to deal with the problem by attempting to reduce expenses. They agreed to manage their finances and develop a family budget designed to (1) meet their basic needs, (2) spend $100 less each month for a total of $1,400, (3) pay an additional $50 each month in rent, and (4) save $50 each month for 1 year for a downpayment on a car.

Having formulated this general strategy, their first task involved determining how they had been spending their money. Average monthly expenses for the last year were calculated from receipts and records. These amounts are given in Table 7-1.

Next, the family needed to distinguish between controllable and uncontrollable expenses; in other words, which monthly expenses could be lowered and which ones could not. For instance, food, clothing, transportation, utilities, personal care, entertainment, and savings are all controllable expenses that can be changed or lowered deliberately on the part of the family. In contrast, rent and insurance are uncontrollable expenses that the

Table 7-1. Family Average Monthly Expenses and Savings Requirements

Expenses	Cost
Rent	$ 400.00
Food	400.00
Clothing	100.00
Transportation	200.00
Utilities	100.00
Insurance	100.00
Personal care	25.00
Entertainment	125.00
Savings	50.00
	Total = $1,500.00

family cannot change. Efforts to reduce expenses must clearly be directed at those areas that can be changed.

After identifying controllable areas, the family discussed ways in which expenses could be cut and developed the monthly budget of $1,400 given in Table 7-2. Compared to their average monthly expenses in the past (Table 7-1), the family planned to reduce spending in five areas: food (from $400 to $350), clothing (from $100 to $75), transportation (from $200 to $175), utilities (from $100 to $75), and entertainment (from $125 to $50). Spending for insurance ($100), personal care ($25), and savings

Table 7-2. Family Monthly Budget

	Cost
Income	$1,400.00
Expenses	
Rent	450.00
Food	350.00
Clothing	75.00
Transportation	175.00
Utilities	75.00
Insurance	100.00
Personal care	25.00
Entertainment	50.00
Total Expenses	$1,300.00
Savings regular	50.00
Saving for car downpayment	50.00
Total Budget	$1,400.00

($50) would remain the same, while rent would be increased from $400 to $450 and an additional $50 each month would be accumulated for the downpayment on the car.

If the family were able to follow this monthly budget plan for a full year, they would be able to meet all of their objectives, including the $600 downpayment for the second car. The challenge, of course, was to adhere to the budgeted amounts each month and thereby avoid significant deviations that could substantially disrupt the family's financial plan and prevent them from attaining their objectives.

In order to monitor adherence to the budget, actual monthly spending should be compared to budgeted spending so that significant deviations could be identified, analyzed, and corrected. An example for the family is given in Table 7-3, comparing budgeted with actual spending. For each category (*i.e.,* rent, food, and so forth) it is possible to determine if the amount spent was different from the amount budgeted. Any difference is referred to as a *variance.*

Reviewing the amounts in Table 7-3, budgeted and actual

Table 7-3.   Comparison of Budgeted and Actual Income and Expenses for First Month

		Budgeted	*Actual*	*Favorable or Unfavorable Variance*
Income		$1,400.00	$1,400.00	$ 0
Expenses				
Rent		$ 450.00	$ 450.00	$ 0.
Food		350.00	375.00	(25.00)
Clothing		75.00	50.00	25.00
Transportation		175.00	175.00	0
Utilities		75.00	100.00	(25.00)
Insurance		100.00	100.00	0
Personal care		25.00	25.00	0
Entertainment		50.00	100.00	(50.00)
	Total expenses	$1,300.00	$1,375.00	$ (75.00)
Excess of income over				$ (75.00)
Expenses		$ 100.00	$ 25.00	$ (75.00)
Savings regular		50.00	50.00	0
Savings for car		50.00	50.00	0
Downpayment		50.00	50.00	0
Savings deficiency		0	(75.00)	(75.00)

( ) = unfavorable variance. Actual expenses exceed budgeted amount.

spending were identical in four categories (rent, transportation, insurance, personal care), and different in four categories (food, clothing, utilities, and entertainment). The variance was unfavorable in three cases (food, utilities, and entertainment), indicating that actual spending exceeded the budgeted amount whereas the opposite was true in one case (clothing). The total variance for the entire budget revealed that the family spent $75 more than was budgeted for that month (the money could have been borrowed or taken from a savings account). Continuation of this pattern would result in a failure to attain family financial objectives.

Consequently, corrective action needs to be directed at the three areas with an unfavorable variance in order to bring actual spending in line with budgeted amounts. Thus, an additional effort is needed to reduce spending on food, clothing, and entertainment. The success of these corrective efforts is measured by comparing actual and budgeted spending for the following months.

If significant or chronic deviations from the budget are not corrected the family's financial objectives will be jeopardized.

In this illustration, the family approached the financial management and budgeting process in a participative manner by obtaining input from all members. This approach significantly increases involvement and enhances acceptance of and commitment to the final budget. All family members perceive partial ownership of the final budget as a function of their participation. Furthermore, feelings of satisfaction, cohesion, and teamwork are fostered. A budget developed in this manner can serve to effectively mobilize and motivate the efforts of everyone concerned.

The need for systematic financial management and budgeting was obvious in this simple example. A well conceived budget generally provides a comprehensive framework for sound financial management. More specifically, a budget accomplishes the following purposes: (1) it supplies a mechanism for translating financial objectives into projected monthly spending patterns, (2) it enhances financial planning and decision making, (3) it clearly identifies controllable and uncontrollable cost areas, (4) it offers a useful format for communicating financial objectives to all concerned parties, (5) it can be used to assign financial responsibility and accountability, (6) it allows for feedback concerning the extent to which actual spending conforms to budgeted spending, (7) it makes possible the early identification of problem areas and thus facilitates the development of effective solutions, and (8) it provides a means of measuring and rewarding financial success.

FINANCIAL MANAGEMENT AND BUDGETING FOR THE HOSPITAL

The situation confronting hospital administrators is similar to the family example just discussed. Hospital administrators find themselves facing a combination of both rising expenses and falling income. For example, the costs to health care institutions of modern technology, medical supplies, new drugs/medicines, and labor have risen dramatically. Unfortunately, several factors have at the same time served to significantly decrease income, including (1) prospective payment systems implemented by the government and many insurance providers, (2) more competition from HMOs, PPOs, and outpatient clinics, and (3) intense pressure from business groups to lower medical costs. These circumstances present a major financial challenge to the health care industry, and nurses must be fully aware of what is occurring in order to respond optimally to the opportunities presented.

The benefits are substantial for those hospitals that react and adapt effectively. If total income exceeds total expenses, institutions will be able to expand services, purchase new equipment, modernize facilities, increase wages and benefits, and offer generally higher quality care and a better working environment. On the other hand, if total income is less than total expenses, hospitals will experience a deficit or loss. Certain consequences typically follow when the problem is severe or becomes chronic. These include cutbacks in staff, reductions in hours worked, decreases in pay and benefits, postponement or cancellation of modernization plans, delays in purchasing new equipment, or reductions in patient services. The quality of patient care often suffers, as well as the quality of work life in the institution. If the financial problems persist, hospitals will eventually go bankrupt and will close down, merge with another stronger organization, or be bought out by a larger health care provider.

People who work in hospitals would clearly prefer to deal effectively with the present financial challenges and ensure that total income exceeds total expenses. Three basic strategies, as discussed in the family example, are required to accomplish this objective: (1) try to increase income, (2) try to decrease expenses, and (3) simultaneously attempt to both increase income and decrease expenses. Most hospital administrators are attempting to follow the third strategy, seeking to boost income, while simultaneously cutting expenses.

Efforts to increase income have included both traditional and nontraditional approaches. For example, many institutions are offering expanded or specialized in-patient services in order to increase occupancy rates. Out-patient clinics are also proliferating, along with a host of health promotion and wellness programs. Nontraditional ventures have included such efforts as the operation of day care and sick child centers, commercial laundry services, and food catering. By combining traditional and nontraditional approaches, hospital administrators hope to ensure that total income exceeds expenses, allowing surplus funds for improvements, expansion, and growth.

While efforts are underway in hospitals in the United States to increase income, most institutions have concentrated more heavily on trying to decrease expenses. Just as in the family example, hospitals must (1) determine what their expenses are, based on past experience, (2) identify controllable cost areas, (3) develop strategies to reduce expenses in those areas, and (4) formulate a budgetary plan to guide, direct, and monitor these efforts.

The implications of such cost-cutting activities for nursing are immediate and significant. First, since nursing costs represent a substantial portion of the overall hospital budget, administrators often tend to focus their attention in this area. Unfortunately, nursing costs are frequently viewed as excessive, in addition to being controllable. Nurses must be prepared consequently to defend their budgetary allocations in the interest of both the quality of patient care and working conditions. Second, nurses must exhibit proactive fiscal responsibility in developing budgets and reducing costs. A thorough, self-examination process can lead to significant cost reductions and can satisfy overall hospital goals. Without such efforts, the intervention of cost control forces external to nursing is inevitable.

Finally, as hospital budgets shrink, interdepartmental competition for dwindling resources will intensify. Success in this competition requires that nurses be intimately familiar with the budgeting process and capable of asserting the importance of their services in economic terms.

With these important thoughts in mind, a simple hospital budgeting example is presented to familiarize nurses with the fundamental concepts involved. There are two basic approaches to developing an organization-wide budget: top-down and bottom-up. In top-down budgeting, senior management develops the complete budget for the hospital as a whole and for all subunits. Thus, for example, a budget would be formulated and given to nursing without the benefit of input from nurses or nurse managers. The problems and shortcomings with such autocratic methods should be obvious.

The preferred option is bottom-up budgeting in which all employees and managers have an opportunity to provide input. As in the family example, such participative approaches foster acceptance, commitment, satisfaction, and motivate performance. In the typical bottom-up method, the hospital's chief financial officer (CFO) provides all managers with projections about future trends and economic conditions that will affect the institution, including such factors as occupancy rates, reimbursement trends, unit supply costs, wages, rates, and inflation rates. Anticipated income is also estimated.

In light of these figures, departmental managers are asked to develop their departmental budgets for the coming year and submit them to their divisional manager for approval. Following this, the hospital's chief executive officer reviews the proposals and then submits them to the board of directors for final approval. Information on a hospital's total patient revenue and expenses for a particular year, along with projections and a budget for the upcoming year, is provided in Table 7-4.

Recall that data for the past year are obtained from actual records of income and spending. Thus, in the preceding year, this hospital generated revenues from patient services totalling 20 million dollars. Overall expenses were 18 million, with a total of 8 million accounted for by the nursing division. A surplus of 2 million dollars was available for much needed new equipment and modernization.

Table 7-4. Hospital Budget Example

Category	Preceding Year	Upcoming Budget Year
Total revenue from patient services	$20,000,000	$18,000,000
Expenses		
Nurses	$ 8,000,000	$ 7,000,000
Radiology	2,000,000	2,000,000
Maintenance	1,500,000	1,100,000
Medical fees and commissions	1,000,000	900,000
Dietary	1,000,000	900,000
Housekeeping	1,000,000	1,000,000
Emergency room	1,000,000	1,000,000
Laboratory	1,000,000	800,000
Utilities	500,000	400,000
Administration	500,000	400,000
Medical records	200,000	200,000
Insurance	200,000	200,000
Financing costs	100,000	100,000
Total expenses	$18,000,000	$16,000,000
Excess of revenue over expenses	$ 2,000,000	$ 2,000,000
Appropriations for new equipment and modernization	$ 2,000,000	$ 2,000,000
Remaining balance	0	0

The figures in the second column in Table 7-4 are based on the projections for the upcoming year. A 10% decrease in revenues is anticipated and thus corresponding reductions in expenses will be attempted without compromising the quality of services provided. As in the family example, not all expenses can be reduced—some are uncontrollable. The costs in this example include insurance and financing costs. Therefore, efforts to reduce costs must be directed at controllable areas and appropriate budgets developed.

The hospital's goal in this example is to meet the projected 10% decrease in patient revenue by cutting expenses in seven areas (nursing, maintenance, medical fees and commissions, dietary, laboratory, utilities, and administration) and still generate a surplus of 2 million dollars to continue modernization efforts. The institutional budget represents a financial framework for reaching these objectives and would be based ideally on extensive collaboration with managers in all departments.

The nursing budget has been reduced from 8 million dollars in the preceding year to a projected 7 million. This figure should be the result of detailed discussions and planning within the nursing division and should not represent a threat to the quality of patient care provided or staff working conditions. In the next section of this chapter, the budget for a medical/surgical unit contained in the nursing division is discussed in more detail to reveal how these challenges can be successfully dealt with.

Just as in the family example, senior hospital administrators monitor financial progress on a monthly basis by comparing budgeted amounts to actual amounts and computing variances. In this manner, potential problem areas can be quickly identified, discussed, and corrected if necessary and units that are doing well can be recognized and rewarded.

FINANCIAL MANAGEMENT AND BUDGETING FOR THE NURSING UNIT

In the preceding section, the hospital administration was confronted with a projected 10% decline in patient revenues. After extensive consultations with all departments, an overall institutional budget was developed to meet the hospital's objectives. The bottom-up budget submitted by the nursing division required a one million dollar reduction in spending from $8,000,000 to $7,000,000. The challenge to nursing managers and staff is to reduce expenses without decreasing care quality. The divisional and unit budgets provide a framework or plan to accomplish this goal. The purpose of this section is to present the financial planning and budgeting process at the level of an individual nursing unit within the nursing division and to illustrate how the system should work and to identify the inherent challenges and opportunities involved.

As in the previous two examples, financial planning and budgeting must begin with a review and identification of past expenses and income for the preceding year in terms of the level of revenue generated by the nursing unit and its expenses. This information will then serve as the basis for making proposed changes in the budget of the upcoming year. Data for a medical/surgical unit for the hospital discussed earlier are provided in Table 7-5. The example is simplified to reflect only expenses

Table 7-5. Nursing Unit Annual Budget Example

Category	Preceding Year	Upcoming Budget Year
Total revenue from patient services	$300,000	$250,000
Expenses		
Nursing division administrative costs	$ 15,000	$ 10,000
Salaries and benefits		
1. Head nurse	50,000	50,000
2. Staff nurses	140,000	125,000
Medical supplies	15,000	12,000
Nonmedical supplies	5,000	3,000
Dietary	7,000	5,500
Linen	3,000	2,000
Equipment rental	3,000	1,500
Equipment maintenance and repair	2,000	2,000
Total expenses	$240,000	$210,000
Excess of revenue over expenses	$ 60,000	$ 40,000

involved in providing patient care and the direct operational expense for the nursing division. Operational expenses incurred by the overall hospital (*i.e.,* administration, financing costs, and insurance) must at some point also be assigned proportionally to the nursing unit as well as the various other revenue-generating centers in the institution.

The total patient revenue and a list of the various expense categories included in the nursing unit budget are outlined in Table 7-5. Before examining these categories individually, it is important to understand the different types of costs and their implications for the budget.

First, costs can be considered as either fixed or variable. Fixed costs are those that remain constant, regardless of fluctuations in patient volume. For example, the head nurse's salary is a cost to the nursing unit that must be paid, regardless of the number of patients cared for. Variable costs, on the other hand, are those that change based on the number of patients serviced. For instance, medical supplies, diet trays, and linen costs vary as a function of patient volume.

Costs can also be classified as direct or indirect. Direct costs are those costs that can be traced specifically to the process of actually providing patient care. These costs include such items as staff salaries and medical supplies. Indirect costs involve factors that cannot be traced easily to the patient care process, such as the costs of nursing division administration, utilities, and maintenance.

A thorough understanding and knowledge of the different types of costs can be invaluable to nurse managers as they attempt to reduce unit expenses. The basic challenge is to identify those cost areas over which the unit can exercise control and then develop strategies to specifically decrease expenses.

Returning to Table 7-5, the information in column one indicates that the nursing unit generated $300,000 in patient revenue for the past year. Expenses totaled $240,000 leaving an excess or surplus of $60,000. Based on projections made by the chief financial officer in consultation with the nursing division, revenue for the upcoming year for this nursing unit is expected to drop by $50,000 to $250,000.

The nursing unit manager and staff are now faced with the challenge of reducing expenses in order to produce a target surplus of $40,000, while continuing to provide high quality patient care. After reviewing past costs and discussing various reduction strategies, the unit decided on the following action plan:

1.   Recommendations were made to and accepted by the nursing vice president to consolidate administrative functions, resulting in a projected savings of $5,000 for the unit. Ordinarily, administrative costs are considered fixed and uncontrollable. Cost-cutting efforts, however, should not overlook the distinct possibility of improving the efficiency of nursing administrative operations and thereby reducing expenses.

2.   Through more effective employee scheduling and a reduction in overtime hours, staff salaries and benefits were to be decreased from $140,000 to $125,000.

3.   More effective supply distribution and utilization strategies were planned to reduce medical supply costs by $3,000, non-medical supply costs by $2,000, and linen costs by $1,000.

4.   Better communication with dietary plans was implemented to reduce mistakes and unused meals and thus cut costs from $7,000 to $5,500.

5.   More efficient planning techniques were introduced to better utilize rented equipment and thus cut expenses by $1,500.

6. Nurses were urged to properly use and maintain equipment in order to decrease contracted maintenance and repair costs.

If the nursing unit successfully implements these strategies, total expenses can be reduced by $30,000 from the preceding year, thus allowing for a $40,000 surplus from total patient revenues of $250,000.

As emphasized earlier, the budget is a plan for monitoring and controlling expenses. Effective use of the budget plan requires monthly reports indicating how well the particular unit is doing. Further investigation and analysis are necessary when discrepancies exist. A simplified report is provided in Table 7-6, indicating budgeted monthly amounts, actual amounts spent, and the variance or difference between the two.

Upon receiving such a report, nurse managers would review the figures and examine the variances. If the actual cost is less than the budgeted amount, the variance is said to be favorable. Actual amounts in excess of budgeted figures are termed *unfavorable variances*. A review of Table 7-6 shows four favorable var-

Table 7-6. Nursing Unit Comparison of Budgeted and Actual Expenses for First Month

Category	Budget	Actual	Favorable or Unfavorable Variance
Revenue	$20,800	$20,800	0
Nursing division administrative costs	$ 800	$ 800	0
Salaries and benefits			
1. Head nurse	4,200	4,200	0
2. Staff	10,415	11,000	$(585)
Medical supplies	1,000	1,100	(100)
Nonmedical supplies	250	150	(100)
Dietary	460	460	0
Linen	170	150	(20)
Equipment rental	125	100	(25)
Equipment maintenance and repair	80	75	(5)
Total expenses	$17,500	$18,035	$(535)
Excess of revenue over expenses	$ 3,300	$ 2,765	$(535)

Monthly budget figures are based on half of the annual budget amounts.

iances (nonmedical supplies, linen, equipment rental, and equipment maintenance and repair) and two unfavorable ones (staff salaries and benefits and medical supplies). Overall, on total patient revenue of $20,800, the unit's expenses were $18,035, leaving a surplus of $2,765, or $535 less than projected.

The favorable variances indicate that the unit has exceeded its goal of reducing expenses in these areas and should continue with its excellent effort. The two unfavorable variances require further investigation regarding the underlying reasons. There are many potential causes of the unfavorable variance in staff salaries and benefits. For example, perhaps several of the unit's nurses were sick in the preceding month, requiring a significant increase in overtime hours. Such events are beyond the control of the unit manager and need only be brought to the attention of superiors to explain the cause. In such situations, one would not expect continued unfavorable variances in the following months.

On the other hand, if the unfavorable variance is a function of poor scheduling by the nurse manager, improvements need to be made in order to keep actual expenses in line with budgeted amounts. Similarly, the unfavorable variance in medical supplies should also be examined and the causes clearly identified and analyzed.

The goals of this monthly budgetary review and evaluation process are ideally to: (1) quickly identify potential problem areas before they get out of control, (2) determine whether problem areas are due to controllable or uncontrollable factors, (3) develop solutions to controllable problems, and (4) recognize and reward nurse managers and staff for delivering quality care within their budget.

RECOMMENDATIONS FOR ACTION

Given the recent changes that have occurred in the health care field, nurses at all levels must possess a fundamental understanding of basic financial planning and budgeting. Such knowledge is essential in capitalizing on the unique opportunities available, competing for financial resources within the health care delivery system, and asserting leadership in improving the cost-effectiveness of the patient care process. With these objectives in mind, the following interrelated recommendations for action are made.

Nursing Education in Preparation

Current nurse managers and staff must be provided with the training and education necessary to familiarize them with the process of financial planning and budgeting. This will require systematic continuing education programs. Madsen and Harper have shown that this can be accomplished successfully with both head nurses and staff.[3] Similar efforts are needed in all hospitals to educate nurses in finance, accounting, fiscal planning and policy, and budgeting.

Although it is important for every nurse to be trained in these areas, it is essential for present and prospective nurse managers. In the absence of informed, educated, and effective nursing leadership, success in dealing with the new financial challenges will be limited. Nurse managers have been selected traditionally more for their clinical skills than for their administrative or financial talent.[3,4] Without deemphasizing the obvious importance of clinical skills, the basic role expectations of nurse managers, as well as staff nurses, must be expanded to include financial skills and expertise.

Continuing education programs are needed to deal with the immediate, short-term problem of providing needed knowledge and skills to presently employed nurses. However, over the long run, nursing preparation programs at the undergraduate and graduate levels must be revised to include more business-related courses in the curriculum. Nursing students must be rigorously and thoroughly prepared to assume their clinical responsibilities within an environment of heightened cost consciousness. The goal of educating the profession in financial matters can be achieved by properly training new nurses and updating current ones.

Budgetary Participation

Nurses must demand an active role in the hospital budgeting process within the framework of a general bottom-up budgeting approach. Nursing staff and managers at all levels should be given the opportunity to participate in developing budgets.

Nurses can no longer allow their budgets to be developed by others outside of the profession.

The American Hospital Association, in the publication entitled, *Managing Under Medicare Prospective Pricing*, strongly recommends that nurses be held accountable for the development, monitoring, and success of their own budgets.[5] This accountability and responsibility are long overdue, given the magnitude and importance of the nursing role in providing patient care. Nurses should demand involvement in the budgetary process and they must be prepared to effectively meet the challenges that follow.

Patient Classification Systems

Many researchers and writers have recognized the importance of formulating more precise patient classification systems in order to more accurately measure the level or intensity of nursing care provided.[6-12] An hour of nursing care is not equivalent across patients with different diagnoses and acuity levels. Continued research is needed in this area, along with the implementation and field testing of new approaches. Required nursing care must be measured accurately and predictably. This will then allow for (1) the clear-cut expression of nursing services in economic terms, (2) more rational and effective planning for nurse staffing, and (3) the objective analysis and improvement of nursing productivity.[2]

Separate Billing for Nursing Care

The importance and cost of nursing care is often obscured by including it in the daily hospitalization charge or room rate. This sad state of affairs must be corrected. Nursing care should be listed as a separate item on the patient's hospital bill.[6,10,11,13,14]

Patients, doctors, health care workers, hospital administrators, and the general public must be educated concerning the vital role that nursing plays in the patient care process. This can be accomplished only by demonstrating the economic cost and value of nursing care. Separate billing would dramatically increase the awareness, recognition, and appreciation of nursing's contribution and would enhance the prestige and power of the profession.

Nursing as a Profit Center

The nursing component of the hospital has been viewed traditionally as an inefficient cost center, unrelated to revenue generation or profit. Nurses must assertively educate hospital administrators and other departments concerning their important role in revenue generation and they must assume the designation as a profit center.[11,15]

By controlling costs and improving efficiency, nursing can exert a major influence on an institution's profit or surplus. This contribution has been overlooked previously and must be emphasized in the future. Furthermore, as a profit center, nurses should be held accountable for their financial performance and should be rewarded accordingly. Legitimate recognition as a revenue-generating activity will significantly improve the respect and appreciation of nurses and their role in the hospital.

The aforementioned interrelated recommendations are intended to serve as a framework for nursing action in the important areas of financial planning and budgeting. Nurses must be adequately prepared to assert their rights, perform effectively, and be held accountable. Success in these endeavors will be invaluable in increasing the importance, power, and prestige of the profession.

SUMMARY AND CONCLUSIONS

1. Nurses must have a fundamental knowledge of the basic concepts involved in financial planning and budgeting in order to respond successfully to the financial challenges in health care.

2. When faced with falling income, in order to remain financially viable, an organization has three basic options: (a) attempt to decrease expenses, (b) attempt to increase income through other means, or (c) simultaneously attempt to both decrease expenses and increase income.

3. A budget is a structured plan for managing income and expenses. Steps in the budgeting process include (a) the identification and analysis of past income and spending levels, (b) the specification of organizational financial objectives, (c) the projection of future income and spending levels necessary to attain organizational goals, (d) the monthly review of actual income and spending levels compared to

budgeted amounts, and (e) the initiation of corrective action in areas where actual spending exceeds budgeted amounts, or actual income falls below projected levels.

4. Within the context of a nursing unit budget, it is important to understand that there are different types of costs involved. Costs, for example, can be considered as either *fixed* or *variable*. Fixed costs are those that remain constant, regardless of fluctuations in patient volume. Variable costs, on the other hand, are those that change as the number of patients changes. Costs can also be classified as either *direct* or *indirect*. Direct costs are those incurred in the process of actually providing individual patient care, whereas indirect costs involve factors not directly traceable to the individual patient.

5. A well formulated budget will accomplish the following major purposes: (a) it supplies a mechanism for translating financial objectives into projected spending patterns, (b) it enhances financial planning and decision making, (c) it offers an effective means of controlling costs, (d) it offers a useful format for communicating financial objectives to all concerned parties, (e) it can be used to clearly assign financial responsibility and accountability, (f) it allows for feedback concerning the extent to which actual spending conforms to budgeted spending, (g) it makes possible the early identification of problem areas and thus facilitates the development of effective solutions, and (h) it provides a means of measuring and rewarding performance.

6. There are two basic approaches to budgeting: top-down and bottom-up. Top-down budgeting involves the formulation of budgets by senior management without the input of employees and managers. Budgets developed in this manner are given to lower level managers for implementation. In bottom-up budgeting, all employees and managers have an opportunity to participate in the process. Bottom-up budgeting is clearly superior to the top-down approach in terms of employee satisfaction, acceptance, commitment, and motivation, and thus it is the preferred method.

7. Hospital administrators are responding to the financial pressures in health care by aggressively attempting to cut costs. A major target of these cost-cutting efforts has been and will continue to be the nursing division. Nurse leaders must be prepared consequently to justify the importance of nursing services in financial terms and defend their budgets to ensure that the quality of patient care remains high.

8. Nursing must take a lead role in demonstrating fiscal responsibility in efforts to control costs in the patient care

process. If these self-improvement efforts are undertaken, it is highly unlikely that forces outside of the profession will attempt to impose control over patient care procedures.

9. The challenge to nursing managers is to identify controllable cost areas, develop specific strategies to reduce expenses, monitor the effectiveness of these strategies, initiate corrective action when necessary, and reward nurses for success.

10. In order to provide nurses with the financial knowledge and skills necessary to succeed in today's changing health care environment, significant continuing education efforts are required for current nurses and basic revisions are needed in programs at the undergraduate and graduate levels to properly prepare future nurses. Furthermore, the fundamental roles of the nurse and nurse manager should be expanded to include financial skills.

11. Nurses must demand an active role in the budgetary process, within the framework of a general bottom-up budgeting approach. Nurses should control the development and monitoring of their own budgets and be held accountable for their financial performance.

12. More research is needed to develop accurate patient classification systems to enable nurses to more precisely measure and predict patient care requirements and express nursing services in economic terms.

13. The cost of nursing care should not be obscured by including it in the daily hospitalization rate or room charge. Nursing care costs should be listed instead as a separate item on a patient's bill.

14. Concerted effort is needed to change the perception that nursing units are simply cost centers. The important role of nursing in revenue generation must be clearly recognized and nursing rightfully identified as a profit center.

Questions for Reflection and Discussion

1. What is a budget and what purposes does it serve?
2. Describe briefly the basic steps in the budgeting process.
3. What is the difference between top-down and bottom-up budgeting? Which is the preferred alternative and why?
4. What can be done at the hospital level to deal with falling revenues from patient care?
5. At the nursing unit level what can be done to deal with falling patient revemues?
6. What is the difference between fixed and variable costs? Give examples of each.

7. What is the difference between direct and indirect costs? Give examples of each.

8. What is the difference between a favorable and unfavorable budget variance? What managerial action should be taken in each case?

9. Why is it important for nursing to be involved in the process of financial planning and budgeting for the hospital?

10. How well prepared are most staff nurses and nurse managers to deal with the emerging financial challenges in health care?

11. What kinds of continuing education programs are needed in nursing to deal effectively with cost-containment pressures?

12. What revisions would you recommend in basic nursing educational programs at the undergraduate and graduate level to better prepare nurses to deal with cost-effectiveness?

13. Why is it important to understand business when dealing with other hospital departments and the administration?

14. Why are accurate patient classification systems so important in costing nursing services and improving productivity?

15. Do you feel that nursing charges should be listed as a separate item on patient hospital bills? Give reasons for your answer.

16. Why are nursing units not typically viewed as profit centers, and what can be done to correct this situation?

17. Should the traditional roles of the nurse and nurse manager be expanded to include expertise in financial matters?

REFERENCES

1. Hoffman F: Financial Management for Nurse Managers. East Norwalk, CT, Appleton–Century–Crofts, 1984
2. Strasen L: Key Business Skills for Nurse Managers. Philadelphia, JB Lippincott, 1987
3. Madsen NL, Harper RW: Improving the nursing climate for cost containment. J Nurs Admin 15(3):11–16, 1985
4. Covaleski MA, Dirsmith MW: Building tents for nursing services through budgeting negotiation skills. Nurs Admin Q 8(2):1–11, 1984
5. American Hospital Association: Managing Under Medicare Prospective Pricing, pp XIII-2. Chicago, AHA, 1983
6. Joel LA: DRG's and RIM's: Implications for nursing. Nurs Outlook 32(1):241–255, 1984
7. Mitchell M, Miller J, Welches L, Walker DD: Determining costs of direct nursing care by DRG's. Nurs Man 15(4):29–32, 1984

8. Riley WJ, Schaefers V: Costing nursing services. Nurs Man 14:40–43, 1983
9. Staley M, Luciano K: Eight steps to costing nursing services. Nurs Man 15:35–38, 1984
10. Thompson JD, Averill RJ, Fetter RB: Planning, budgeting, and controlling—one look at the future: Case mix cost accounting. Health Services Res 14(2):111–125, 1979
11. Thompson JD, Diers D: DRG's and nursing intensity, Nurs Health Care 6(8):435–439, 1985
12. Walker DD: The cost of nursing care in hospitals. In Aiken L (ed): Nursing in the 80's. Philadelphia, JB Lippincott, 1982
13. Laurer EB: Where will the money go? Economic forecasting and nursing's future. Nurs Health Care 6(3):132–135, 1986
14. Olsen SM: The challenges of prospective pricing: Work smarter. J Nurs Admin 14(4):22–26, 1984
15. Riley WJ, Schaefers V: Nursing operations as a profit center. Nurs Man 15:43–46, 1984

8

Efficiently Controlling
Use of Supplies

THE DOUBLE digit inflation rate of recent health care costs in the United States is familiar to anyone in the nursing profession. A major component of these rising costs has been the dramatic increase in the price of medical supplies. Smith has estimated that many hospitals spend 40% or more of their total budget on supplies alone.[1] Consequently, if supply prices are rising rapidly, this will contribute to an overall increase in the cost of health care.

Many of the more expensive supply items are those used by nurses in providing high quality patient care. The increasing cost of these items can be traced to two primary factors. First, as medical care has become more sophisticated and complex, the supplies needed to provide and support that care have become more expensive. Second, the use of disposable items has also contributed to the overall increase in supply costs.

The purpose of this chapter is to examine the issue of the use of supplies from a nursing perspective. It should be emphasized that the use of medical supplies is an area over which nurses exert a great deal of discretionary control. Thus, cost-efficient utilization of the supplies used in providing patient care is a nursing responsibility.

Unfortunately, considerable anecdotal evidence exists which suggests that nursing supplies are often used in an inappropriate, inefficient, and wasteful manner. The dimensions of this potentially significant problem are addressed, along with promising solutions. Actual nursing examples are used to illustrate the specific kinds of problems that exist and the innovative solutions to solve them.

NATURE AND EXTENT OF THE PROBLEM

Smith has indicated that approximately 42% of the average hospital budget is spent on supplies.[1] Typically, two thirds of that amount comprises medically oriented supplies, for which usage patterns are influenced significantly by nursing.

Accurate statistics on the extent to which medical supplies are misused in the patient care process are largely unavailable. In the past, supply use practices have rarely been monitored systematically and thus the magnitude of any problems cannot be determined precisely. However, based on extensive interviews, interactive seminars, and conversations with nurses and nurse administrators, a potentially serious and expensive problem has emerged. When asked to cite examples of inappropriate use of supplies, an inordinate number of responses has been typically received. In this section, a sample of these incidents is presented to illustrate the nature and possible extent of this general problem. Regrettably, summary figures concerning the frequency of misuse or the overall monetary value are unavailable, but can only be estimated from the examples provided.

How serious this potential problem is in your unit or hospital will require careful investigation and analysis. The collection of anecdotal data assembled suggests that the misuse of supplies is a significant problem in many nursing units and these amounts probably represent only the "tip of the iceberg" with respect to the overall problem. Thus, this area should receive the attention of all nurses and nurse administrators concerned with improving the cost efficiency of the patient care process.

Actual examples of cost-inefficient use of supplies given by nurses from several hospitals include the following:

1. Intravenous items in one hospital were stored in a box in the patient unit, with nurses responsible for attributing the cost of these supplies to patients as they were used. Unfortunately, the charges were frequently not made, resulting in an annual cost to the unit of $2,000.00 for these items alone.

2. On one nursing unit, 4×3 sponges were used to cleanse wounds as opposed to equally effective cotton balls. The sponges cost 90 cents each, whereas the cotton balls cost less than 50 cents for 100.

3. In one hospital, nurses often opened sealed admission packets to get the pencil inside for report writing, discarding the rest of the contents.

4. A frequently cited example involved the widespread misuse of chux to clean up spills and messes instead of a mop. Chux in one hospital cost 66 cents each, thus representing an unnecessarily expensive cleaning method.

5. One nursing unit reported a common practice of opening suture kits to get the scissors inside and then discarding the remainder of the contents.

6. Another frequently mentioned illustration of the misuse of supplies involved the misuse of hospital forms for scratch paper and report writing. Printed forms cost substantially more than plain or scratch paper. For example, in one institution, charting forms cost 7 cents each. Casual misuse of these forms on a regular basis could become an expensive problem.

7. In one hospital, shaving kit packets cost $18.50 each, and they could be reused for more than 1 day for shaving male patients. The common practice, however, was to use a new kit daily and then to dispose of it, resulting in a weekly cost of $129.50 for shaving.

8. The failure to transfer all supplies in the room when a patient is moved was a common problem reported in one hospital, resulting in excessive and unnecessary use of supplies.

9. The problem of petty or casual theft is experienced by most hospitals. Items commonly targeted include alcohol wipes, tape, pens, pencils, paper, and penlites. Rarely, however, do hospitals or nursing units accurately monitor and measure this problem in order to determine its magnitude and overall cost.

10. Finally, Huey suggests that many common patient care procedures result in the clinically unnecessary use of supplies.[2] As an example, she cites the generally accepted practice of

changing intravenous (IV) tubing every 24 hours despite extensive evidence collected by the Center for Disease Control indicating that doing this every 48 hours is clinically acceptable and is certainly less costly.

These examples and many others suggest that the misuse of supplies is a common practice in most nursing units. Given the rising cost of medical supplies used in providing patient care, the total monetary losses attributable to this problem are potentially enormous. The importance of this topic necessitates thoughtful attention and concerted action from all nurses.

ORIGINS OF THE PROBLEM

The general problem of inefficient use of supplies by nurses probably has several interrelated causes. A number of these potentially significant factors are introduced in this section.

1. Perhaps the most important cause is a lack of recognition and awareness of the problem and its magnitude on the part of hospital administrators, nurse managers, and staff nurses. Typically, the issue of efficient use of supplies has not received a great deal of attention within hospital settings. Consequently, most nurses are not fully aware of this potentially costly problem and its impact on costs. Indicative of this mode of thinking is an article by Harrell and Frauman,[3] in which they state that "supplies are not major hospital expenditures."

2. Compounding the impact of the first factor is the traditional mode of providing patient care practiced within the former retrospective payment system. Nursing care has historically been provided without major concern for the volume or manner in which supplies were used. Old habits and traditional practices are difficult to change and thus contribute to the continuing costly problem of the misuse of supplies.

3. Another related cause of the overall problem centers on the nurse's lack of knowledge concerning the cost of supplies used in providing patient care. In an exercise (see p 203) that requires an estimate of the cost of commonly used supplies, nurses significantly underestimated the cost in over 80% of all cases. Without an accurate understanding and clear knowledge of the cost of supplies, the monetary impact of misuse problems cannot be appreciated and the perceived need to improve will not be strong.

4. Given that nursing has not generally recognized the impor-

tance of the supply misuse issue, it is not surprising to find that individual nurses are typically unfamiliar with the basic concepts and techniques of efficient use of supplies. Unfortunately, this type of information has not been included traditionally in nursing educational programs at any level. Without a rudimentary understanding of the basic issues involved in the use of supplies and some of the strategies for improving efficiency, significant progress in dealing with this problem will be elusive.

5. Another possible reason for the problem of a misuse of supplies concerns the lack of incentives to reinforce and reward good performance. Nursing units that save money in their supply budget frequently discover that the money is returned to the hospital general fund, and their future budget is reduced accordingly. This practice serves as a lack of incentive to use supplies more efficiently. If improvements are desired, functional incentive systems must be developed to measure and reward desirable performance. This issue is more fully discussed in Chapter 13.

6. Although the first five potentially important determinants of the problem of misuse of supplies are related to underlying characteristics of the health care and educational systems in the United States, this discussion would be incomplete without addressing factors at the level of the individual nurse. Thus, a sixth possible factor involves nursing attitudes toward efficient use of supplies. In many cases, these attitudes are less than positive, with nurses believing that it is not their responsibility to pay attention to such trivial and materialistic matters. Many nurses believe instead that providing top quality patient care is their only responsibility, without regard to the amount or manner in which supplies are used. Such attitudes are no longer functional in the evolving health care system. Quality care must continue to be provided, but as efficiently as possible. This necessarily includes close scrutiny of the way in which nursing supplies are used.

7. Another important individual level variable involves poor planning on the part of the staff nurse. A lack of proper and accurate care planning can easily result in the misuse of supplies in the form of (a) not enough of a particular item to perform a required procedure, (b) too much of a particular item, (c) the wrong item, leading to inappropriate use of another item, and (d) forgetting a required item, resulting in unnecessary delays or unconventional, cost inefficient substitutions.

8. Finally, the interview data collected from nurses and nurse

managers suggest that laziness is often a cause of poor use of supplies. Rather than looking for or obtaining the appropriate item, nurses occasionally make do with a more convenient, yet expensive alternative. As mentioned in the earlier examples, rather than looking for a pair of scissors, nurses have obtained one from an available suture kit and discarded the remainder of the contents. Many factors contribute to such behavior — a lack of awareness of the costs involved, perhaps a poor attitude, or poor planning — but the fundamental issue is a lack of proper work motivation.

The general problem of inefficient use of supplies probably has several interrelated and powerful causes that, when combined, present nursing with a difficult challenge. Effectively solving this problem requires an examination of the potential causes within a particular hospital and the development of an improvement strategy designed to specifically address the problems. In the next section, a general approach to correcting the misuse of supplies is presented.

SIX-STEP CORRECTIVE PROGRAM

The problem of inefficient use of supplies is one that is commonly encountered in the private sector. When income or sales are down, businesses typically cut their own costs by reducing the size of their labor force or by improving the efficiency of supply or material use. Consequently, a great deal of knowledge has been accumulated concerning the ingredients of a successful program to improve the practices involving the use of supplies.

In this section, a comprehensive six-step corrective program is presented. The six steps include (1) education and awareness, (2) problem identification, definition, and measurement, (3) participative solution development and goal setting, (4) solution implementation, (5) solution evaluation and revision, and (6) incentives for goal attainment. When available, examples in nursing are used to illustrate how the program should ideally function.

Step 1. Education and Awareness

As mentioned earlier, an important likely reason for misuse of supplies in nursing centers on the lack of understanding and awareness of the nature and magnitude of the problem and the cost of items commonly used in providing patient care. Thus, a necessary first step in rectifying the problem is to educate nurses and make them aware of the importance and cost magnitude of the misuse of supplies. Without this basic understanding and knowledge, significant and lasting improvement is impossible.

The importance of this first step cannot be overestimated. Experience has shown that in many situations, the misuse problem can be reduced substantially by educating nurses about the basic issues and costs involved. Responsible and concerned nurses typically respond favorably to educational programs, often resulting in immediate and significant improvements in supply use practices.

Various specific approaches are available to accomplish the desired educational objectives. Four of the more effective and innovative ones are briefly presented.

SMALL GROUP DISCUSSIONS

A particularly effective approach involves introducing the general problem in a nonthreatening manner to small groups of nurses (*e.g.,* at the unit level) and generating a discussion of the key issues involved. For instance, nurses can be asked to offer examples of supply misuse that they may be familiar with and identify the consequences of such problems for themselves, the unit, and the hospital. A discussion of the possible causes of these problems can also be enlightening.

The discussion leader can be the head nurse or unit director, someone from staff development, a member of the nursing administration, or an outside consultant. One should realize that the success of this strategy depends largely on the expertise of this person. The discussion leader must be nondirective and must encourage the participation of all nurses in the group. Rather than lecturing about the topic, use of the Socratic method tends to be more appropriate. This involves formulating key questions for the group to guide the discussion and allow the nurses to discover and generate the basic dimensions of the problem on their own.

Examples of specific questions that can be helpful include (a) Is anyone familiar with a specific situation in which nursing supplies were used in a less than optimal or efficient manner?, (b) How much do you think instances of misuse of supplies cost the unit, and over a 1-year period, what do these costs add up to?, (c) How does this problem affect the hospital, the unit, and you personally?, (d) Why do you think we have problems with inefficient use of supplies in nursing?, and (e) Do most nurses know how much patient care supplies cost?

If done properly, phrasing questions in this manner will elicit active participation and will allow nurses to explore the basic dimensions of the issue and realize that the problem is a nursing responsibility. A logical continuation of this group process involves mobilizing members to generate problem solutions (Step 3 in the corrective approach). However, after educating nurses as to the basic issues in cost-effectiveness, it is first necessary to identify, measure, and cost out major supply use problems. This is discussed later in Step 2 of the corrective program.

PRICE IS RIGHT GAME

An entertaining yet effective approach to demonstrating that nurses are generally unfamiliar with supply costs is to play a modified version of The Price is Right. This game has been developed and successfully used by Brenda Terrell, the Director of Educational Services for the Methodist Hospitals in Gary, Indiana.

The game involves dividing a group of nurses into two teams from which representatives are chosen to play each round. Team representatives are asked to estimate the cost of commonly used patient care items that are shown to everyone and are then briefly discussed. Other team members are allowed to offer suggestions to their representative in reaching an estimate. The teams take turns giving the final estimate and the team that comes closest to the actual price is given a small prize. The team with the highest score at the end of the game is also given a small prize. Typically, 50 to 20 items are used. A list of sample items is provided in Table 8-1. As mentioned earlier, nursing estimates are lower than actual item costs in over 80% of all cases, which dramatically illustrates the point that nurses are often unaware of supply costs and do not appreciate how expensive they are.

The Price is Right is an excellent vehicle to generate interest, participation, and enthusiasm, while at the same time emphasizing an important point. Participants in this game are often amazed at their lack of knowledge and are generally convinced of

Table 8-1. Sample Nursing Supplies Used in "Price is Right" Exercise

Item	Estimated Cost	Actual Cost
1. 1000 cc lactate		
2. 1000 cc 5% glucose		
3. Chux		
4. Enema kit		
5. Jackson Pratt 100 cc catheter		
6. IVAC probe		
7. Sterile closed drainage bag		
8. Foley catheter		
9. 24-hour disposable collection bottle		
10. Trach care set		

the need for some method of accurately communicating supply costs to all nurses.

POSTED SUPPLY COST LISTS

A straightforward and useful approach to communicating supply costs to nurses is to prominently display a list of the most commonly used supplies and their associated costs on the unit bulletin board. Nurses should be encouraged to familiarize themselves with the data on the listing and any changes can be emphasized at unit meetings.

Given typical space limitations, only the top 25 supply items (in terms of usage) should be posted. However, a complete and current price list of all supplies used in the patient care process should be readily available to nurses for consultation. Unfortunately, few hospitals provide such information to nurses. However, accurate knowledge of these costs is a necessary first step in improving supply use practices and in reducing expenditures.

ITEM PRICE STICKERS

A fourth approach to educating nurses about supply costs involves placing price stickers on individual items, when practical. For instance, it would be ridiculous to try to put stickers on individual cotton balls! Yet for most items employed in the patient care process, the use of price stickers is feasible. Not only does this system provide direct, immediate, and accurate information to nurses about supply costs, but it also facilitates the process of charging items to individual patients.

A rational plan for the use of stickers involves the following guidelines in selecting items to be stickered: (a) those that are most expensive, (b) those that are used most frequently, (c) those that are most frequently forgotten in the charging process, and (d) those that can be individually stickered. Thus, all patient care items need not be stickered in order for such a program to be effective in reducing supply costs *and* minimizing lost charges.

In all instances, the fundamental objectives of the methods discussed are the same: (a) to introduce nurses to the problem of the misuse of supplies, (b) to emphasize the cost magnitude of the problem, and (c) to communicate the cost of specific supplies used in providing patient care. Many other procedures are available to accomplish these objectives, and new approaches are being developed around the country, limited only by the ingenuity and creativity of nurses.

Nurses must view this problem as their own responsibility and take bold steps to develop innovative solutions. The critical first step must involve improving education and awareness. If properly done, significant improvement can result from the enhanced knowledge and appreciation of the problem and its consequences.

Step 2. Problem Identification, Definition, and Measurement

Once nurses understand the basic issue of the misuse of supplies and its consequences, they must focus on specific problem areas confronting a particular nursing unit or hospital. Although similarities do exist, no two nursing units or hospitals are alike in the way in which they use supplies. Practices differ significantly, and what may be a major problem in one unit, is nonexistent in another.

Consequently, in Step 2, a thorough review of supply use practices and potential problem areas in each individual unit is highly recommended. This process is best accomplished in a participative manner by involving staff nurses in the evaluation of common supply use practices and identification of possible problems.

After specific problems have been identified, they should be defined clearly and priced. The pricing process involves estimating the frequency of occurrence of a particular problem and multiplying it by the cost of the supply item being used. For instance, using an example cited earlier concerning shaving kits (which cost $18.50 each), if kits can be used for 1 week in shaving patients, but are used typically on a daily basis, the extra cost is $129.50 (7 days) — $18.50, or $111.00 per week. Were this to occur with an average of ten male patients per week in a nursing unit, the total cost is $1,110.00 on a weekly basis. When dealing with prospective payment systems, this additional cost represents a real loss in income to the hospital.

All potentially important problem areas should be priced in a similar manner. This then allows for prioritization of the various misuse practices in terms of their cost impact. Attention should be directed at that point to addressing those problems with the highest cost to the unit or hospital. Thus, rather than spending time with trivial problems, the most serious ones can be dealt with first.

Smith has estimated that the top 10% of hospital supply items in terms of their cost typically account for over 70% of total supply expenditures.[1] The same is probably true of the supply misuse problem. The top 10% of a unit's specific supply misuse practices will probably account for 70% of the costs of the overall problem. Corrective attention should therefore be focused on the most salient problem areas first.

In the second step of the corrective program, the basic objective is to carefully identify possible problem areas, measure and price their impact, and select for immediate attention those areas with the highest cost. This process should be completed before proceeding to the third step.

Step 3. Participative Solution Development and Goal Setting

Once a nursing unit or hospital has identified its major supply misuse problems, the next step involves the participative development of a solution and the setting of target goals. Active participation in the solution development is recommended for several reasons, such as: (a) the involvement of those people, staff nurses, who are most familiar with the problems and thus the ultimate solutions, (b) the synergy resulting from the participative group process can often result in creative, high-quality solutions, (c) acceptance of group-generated solutions is improved through the perception of ownership, and (d) commitment to group solutions is enhanced, also through the process of perceived ownership.

Once solutions have been generated, it is then necessary to establish specific target goals for reducing problem frequency and cost. These goals will serve to motivate and direct behavior and act as a yardstick to measure progress in solving a particular problem. The goal setting process is described in more detail in Chapter 7.

As emphasized throughout this chapter, the misuse of supplies is a responsibility of nurses. Thus, it is necessary for nurses to attack this often costly problem and develop nursing-based solutions. This process is already underway in nursing units and hospitals in the United States. Some examples of problems encountered and the innovative solutions that have been developed by creative nurses are provided below.

Problem: High Cost of Disposable Items. As mentioned earlier, one of the major factors contributing to the rapid increase in supply expenditures has been the shift to expensive disposable patient care items. Many hospitals are attempting to deal with this growing problem by reevaluating the merits and relative cost of potentially reusable items.

Martin reported on the conclusions of an international conference dealing with the reuse of disposable medical devices, sponsored by the Institute for Health Policy Analysis at the Georgetown University Medical Center.[4] The conference attracted leading professionals from nursing, medicine, and hospital administration, in addition to manufacturer representatives. Among the more significant findings were the following:

(a) Reuse of "disposable" items is an extensive, though unpublicized practice.

(b) Improved cost-effectiveness is not evident in all cases.

(c) The issue should be openly and publicly addressed.

(d) Research is needed to determine strict quality control procedures and protocols.

(e) Comparative studies are needed to determine the relative cost-effectiveness of reusing "disposable" items.

(f) A clearing house to share research findings and practices should be established.

The safe and cost efficient reuse of previously categorized single use items is clearly possible. Nursing should continue to take a leading role in examining the potential application of this practice and establish strict guidelines for sterilization protocols. The quality of patient care cannot be sacrificed or jeopardized. However, where clinically sound item reuse is possible, controlled studies should be done to carefully examine the potential cost savings.

As Martin and Martin, Campbell, Dowler, and Palmer have asserted, the costs of handling and sterilization are sometimes greater than the potential savings resulting from reuse.[4-6] The only way to adequately address this issue is to conduct the necessary comparative research. With particularly expensive items, significant cost savings will possibly occur when clinically sound reuse practices are implemented.

Problem: Theft of Medical Supplies. One hospital had been experiencing a chronic problem with the theft of commonly used nursing supplies, such as alcohol wipes, tape, pens, pencils, paper, and penlites. Although involving relatively inexpensive items, the theft frequency was high enough that the overall problem was costing thousands of dollars each year.

The nursing division suggested a solution — an in-house, hospital operated store to sell various medical supplies to employees at slightly above cost. Items to be sold included those that were common targets for pilferage, along with other supplies recommended by the nursing staff. Controlled or technically sophisticated medical items, of course, such as syringes or IV tubing, were not sold. Prices were set slightly higher than the hospital's cost in order to cover operating expenses, in much the same way as a cafeteria or pharmacy, in which employees typically receive major discounts.

The supply store concept was combined with three other components. First, an educational program was given to all staff members, emphasizing the theft problem and the monetary costs to the hospital. The issue of "casual" theft was explicitly addressed and identified as a major drainage of hospital finances. In addition, the responsibility of every employee not to steal and to report observed violations by others was emphasized.

Second, a new policy of increased monitoring of supply use practices, to include potential theft, was announced. Finally, individuals who were caught stealing were punished. The first offense was punished by suspension and the second offense was punished by dismissal.

The thrust of this four component program was to provide major deterrents for stealing and to encourage people to be honest. Although no exact figures were available from the hospital, monetary losses attributable to employee theft dropped dramatically once the program was implemented. Thus, this approach represents a promising potential solution to the problem of employee theft of medical supplies.

Problem: Clinically Unnecessary and Expensive Patient Care Practices. As mentioned earlier, Huey has argued that many common patient care procedures are clinically unnecessary and result in needless additional supply expenditures.[2] To illustrate her point, she notes the widespread practice of changing IV tubing every 24 hours. The Center for Disease Control has collected data on this issue and now recommends that changes every 48 hours are clinically acceptable, and certainly less expensive.

Nursing must begin to systematically reassess the patient care process in light of the new imperatives for cost-effectiveness. As Huey indicates, significant cost savings are often possible without sacrificing the quality of patient care. A key question for nursing has become, how to provide high quality patient care while using medical supplies as efficiently as possible. Rigorous clinical evaluations of new alternative care procedures is required. When research results indicate that care quality remains high, while costs are reduced, the new procedure should be adopted.

Problem: Lost Patient Charges for Supply Items. A major problem facing many hospitals is the loss of revenues resulting from a failure by nurses to properly charge individual patients for supplies used in providing their care. Numerous reasons for this problem exist and several potential solutions have been proposed, including the previously discussed practice of putting individual price stickers on all chargeable items.

One of the most promising, innovative, and comprehensive solutions that has been offered is presented in an article by

Crookston and Kirchhoff.[7] Their approach essentially involves the use of a single page charge sheet, listing medical supplies commonly needed in providing patient care, with spaces to write in other items not listed. This newly designed charge sheet is intended for use with a single patient over a 24-hour period. A tally mark is placed next to the appropriate item on the list as supplies are used. Separate columns are provided for each of the three nursing shifts, along with the total for all shifts.

The responsible nurse on each shift completes the charge sheet and signs it. One copy of the final document is sent to the central storeroom for inventory control purposes and one copy is retained with the patient's chart.

This system has been implemented successfully and used at the University of Utah Hospital in Salt Lake City, Utah. It provides a simple, straightforward, comprehensive, and easy-to-use approach to accurately record patient supply charges. Responsibility and accountability are assigned to the principal nurse providing the care for each patient. This system, along with the simplicity of recording tally marks next to the items used, acts to encourage nurses to accurately record their use of supplies.

The new charge system developed by Crookston and Kirchhoff has a great deal to recommend it and cogently demonstrated that intelligent, creative nurses are eminently and uniquely qualified to solve the cost-effectiveness problems facing the profession.[7]

Problem: Opening Admission Kits for Pencils. One hospital has experienced a persistent problem that involved nurses opening patient admission kits in order to obtain the pencil inside and then discarding the remaining contents. This senseless and expensive practice was curtailed with a simple nursing-based solution.

All staff nurses were issued clip boards with pencils attached by a flexible cord to a ring at the top. This prevented the pencils from being misplaced easily or lost. When combined with an announcement at unit meetings of the cost involved in opening admission kits for pencils, the new strategy eliminated that troublesome problem.

The aforementioned problems and potential solutions provide actual examples of how nurses are dealing boldly and effectively with the supply misuse issue. Further effort, initiative, and creativity are needed to continue to successfully attack these problems.

Step 4. Solution Implementation

Once a nursing unit or hospital has developed potentially effective solutions to their salient supply misuse problems, it is then necessary to mobilize and organize the resources required to successfully implement a particular solution. This entails communicating to all parties involved the purpose and nature of the new program and their specific roles. For example, a new charging system, similar to the one described earlier, would require the active involvement and commitment of the central supply room management and staff.

The ultimate success of any program designed to improve supply use practices depends on the active support of everyone involved. The nursing manager must ensure that this critical support is obtained and that the requisite tangible resources (*e.g.,* additional funds, new equipment) are also available for effective implementation.

Step 5. Solution Evaluation and Revision

Ideally, during the process of developing solutions to supply misuse problems, setting goals, and planning implementation, attention should be directed toward devising a system to monitor the impact of the proposed solutions. If a program has been developed to reduce lost charges, a procedure to systematically monitor and measure lost charges should be formulated. Only in this manner is it possible to determine if a particular strategy is working to reduce costs.

By monitoring the consequences of a corrective program, potential problem areas can be identified and quickly rectified. As is the case with most plans, unanticipated problems often result, requiring modifications to ensure success.

From a motivational perspective, measuring and periodically publicizing or posting the results of the monitoring process can serve as a tremendous reinforcer and incentive. When nurses have expended considerable time and energy in implementing a corrective strategy, solid evidence indicating that the program is working has a positive motivational impact.

In summary, a good measuring and monitoring system will allow one to (a) determine if a proposed solution to a supply misuse problem is working as intended, (b) identify malfunctioning approaches quickly and initiate necessary modifications, and (c) reinforce the efforts of nurses and motivate continued commitment.

Step 6. Incentives for Goal Attainment

A major point made in Chapter 13 is that people generally respond well to incentives in the workplace. Consequently, if more cost-effective supply use practices are desired, powerful incentives must be found to motivate and encourage appropriate behaviors. Although this topic is covered more fully in Chapter 13, two key aspects of incentives as they relate to the supply use problem are discussed here.

First, in many hospitals, strong deterrents exist and serve to actively discourage cost-effective use of supplies. For example, the "reward" for saving money in a unit supply budget often entails (a) returning those savings to the hospital's general fund, and (b) reducing the unit's supply budget for the following year by the amount saved.

The motivational consequences of such actions should be obvious. For the head nurse and staff nurses who worked hard to reduce supply expenditures, these outcomes constitute a real form of punishment, thus discouraging similar future cost-effective behaviors. The continuation of such ill-conceived administrative practices is clearly dysfunctional. Positive incentives must be identified and linked explicitly to success in reducing unit supply costs. Ideally, information concerning these performance–reward contingencies should be disseminated to all nurses prior to actually beginning a cost-containment program. In this way, the motivational potential of the available incentive is maximized.

The second key point concerns the type of incentives offered to nurses. Considerable research has shown that nonmonetary rewards (*e.g.,* formal recognition programs and paid time off) can serve as a powerful incentive for many people. However, with respect to the issue of cost-effective use of supplies, a reliance on nonmonetary rewards alone is probably insufficient to motivate the desired behaviors.

Given that management is exhorting nurses to save money

through more efficient use of supplies, it only seems fair that some percentage of the total saving should be distributed to the nurses involved. Private industry has long used this type of incentive plan to encourage cost-cutting behaviors, and a growing number of progressive hospitals are beginning to follow suit.[8] People do respond to incentives and money is more often than not perceived as a valued reward. Thus, it would seem advisable to use monetary incentives to promote cost-effective use of supplies by offering a percentage of the total monetary savings to the participating nurses in the form of a pay bonus.

The six step corrective program represents a systematic approach to dealing with the costly problem of the misuse of supplies. Following the procedures outlined in the program should result in significant reductions in the frequency of specific misuse practices and the magnitude of total supply expenditures.

TWO RELATED ISSUES—
SUPPLY PROCUREMENT AND STORAGE

When considering nursing use of supplies, two closely related issues should also be addressed: supply procurement and supply storage. *Procurement* refers to the process of obtaining or ordering supplies, whereas *storage* involves the general function of inventory management and specific procedures for ensuring that medical supplies are available to nurses when needed. Both procurement and storage practices have important implications for the overall cost-effectiveness of nursing use of supplies. In this section, potentially serious and expensive problems in these two areas are discussed, along with proposed solutions.

Supply Procurement

The process of obtaining the medical supplies needed to provide high quality patient care is more involved and complicated than most nurses would imagine. Improper, inefficient procurement practices can create significant and costly problems for nursing. Smith and Eusebio, Louisignau, Horger–Scheuber, and Jorlett have investigated these issues and concluded that the following are major potential problems associated with poor procurement practices[1,9]:

  1. A lack of adequate nursing input into procurement decisions often results in products that fail to meet clinical nursing requirements.

2. Improper or insufficient product testing leads frequently to the procurement of products that do not function as expected or required.

3. A lack of standardization in ordering the same product for all units in a hospital can result in a host of specific problems: (a) individual units place small product orders with manufacturers, resulting in higher product prices, (b) inventory requirements are increased by the need to stock small amounts of several different products that perform the same function, (c) training and product orientation costs are increased due to the needs for specialized sessions for each product, and (d) nursing transfers within the hospital are complicated by the use of different products on each unit.

These and other similar problems combine to make improper, inefficient procurement a practice that nurses can no longer tolerate or afford. Effective solutions are relatively straightforward given the nature of the specific problem areas. Perhaps the most comprehensive approach to the product review and ordering process is offered by Smith,[1] in which she details a ten-step procedure designed to correct the problems discussed and efficiently supply nurses with the medical products needed to provide consistent high quality care.

The potential monetary savings attributable to improved procurement practices were estimated by Eusebio and associates.[9] In their study, the adoption of standardized products throughout the target hospital allowed for simplifying the procurement process and ordering products in larger quantities, thus lowering individual product costs. The overall savings to the hospital resulting from the new procedures in a 1 year period were $100,000.00. Given the widespread lack of efficient procurement policies, similar savings are likely to occur in many hospitals when improvements are made. Based on the available literature in both business management and nursing, some of the more useful and promising procurement practices recommended to improve the success and cost-effectiveness of the process include the following:

1. Strong, assertive nursing input into procurement decisions involving products used in the patient care process is a necessity. Since nurses are the primary users of many of

these items, their evaluations are essential in ensuring that clinical requirements are met.

2. Within a division or department of nursing Eusebio and associates recommend that one person be assigned the primary responsibility for coordinating all nursing procurement activities,[9] to include (a) representing nursing on hospital-wide procurement committees, (b) soliciting product recommendations from the nursing staff, (c) identifying product needs and developing specifications, (d) planning and directing clinical tests of new products, (e) coordinating in-service product orientation sessions, and (f) representing the nursing department to all manufacturers' representatives. Given the growing importance of efficient use of supplies, it would seem prudent to have one person in charge of this critical area on a full-time basis.

3. Controlled clinical tests of all new supply items are recommended to substantiate and verify manufacturers' claims and fully evaluate a product's performance within the patient care context. These tests should be made under the direction of nursing personnel to ensure that the product meets all essential clinical requirements.

4. A concerted effort should be made to standardize product usage across all nursing units within a hospital. The advantages of using the same product to accomplish a particular purpose, as opposed to multiple similar products, are overwhelming. Nurses must work to achieve the consensus needed to make standardized product use function effectively in all units.

5. Once a standardized product has been identified, manufacturers who offer that particular product which also meets the hospital's specifications, should be invited to bid on the order. Product orders will tend to be larger with standardization, thus qualifying for volume discounts. Especially when expensive orders are involved, nurses should encourage competition between manufacturers and they should work with them to obtain the best possible overall package, to include price, warranty, service, and in-house orientations. If a manufacturer is genuinely interested in the order, the company will generally be willing to compromise and include extra features to obtain a large contract. Such practices are common in the business world and should be systematically exploited by nurses in seeking the best deal for their money.

Product procurement is an important component in the overall supply use process. Unfortunately, procurement procedures are often inefficient and unsuccessful. Nurses can and should make a difference in improving this situation. Following the guidelines offered in this section can result in large savings in cost and can significantly enhance effectiveness.

Supply Storage

The storage of medical items needed in the patient care process is an important factor affecting the overall efficiency of supply use systems. As Shukla has pointed out, the major objective from a nursing perspective is to design supply storage systems and procedures to maximize effectiveness and time spent in direct patient care, while minimizing costs.[10]

Supply storage falls under the general heading of inventory management — a process that any business must master in order to obtain long-term success. The basic challenge in inventory management is to keep the appropriate amount of supplies, materials, and products available. Major difficulties arise when too much or too little inventory is maintained.

Business in the United States has traditionally done a poor job in managing inventory, typically believing that "more is better." International competition and Japanese management techniques have influenced American business to introduce several improvements in this area, which can be applied easily in hospital settings. Before discussing these improvement strategies, the major potential obstacles confronting sound inventory management are discussed. As mentioned above, difficulties typically arise when not enough or too much inventory is kept available. This is readily apparent when considering the nursing role in providing patient care. For example, specific problems associated with not enough inventory in a nursing unit (*i.e.,* the situation when supplies needed in the patient care process are not adequately stocked or available in the unit) include (a) gross misuse of valuable nursing time spent in looking for or obtaining the necessary items, (b) possible misuse of supplies substituted for missing items, (c) increased levels of frustration and stress and lower job satisfaction, and perhaps most important, (d) potentially serious, and in some emergency cases, even life-threatening lapses in quality patient care. Given the importance and severity of these problems, adequate, readily accessible levels of needed supplies must be maintained in all units.

The immediate and personal impact of these issues on individual staff nurses is substantial: it often interferes with their effectiveness and creates feelings of frustration, stress, dissatisfaction, and inadequacy. Consequently, many nurses have taken informal steps to correct the situation by maintaining "secret supplies" of commonly used or critical items. In one hospital, an inspection of these hidden items revealed that overall unit inventories were, on average, two times larger than those required to operate effectively. In other words, when all of the "secret supplies" were combined with those kept for general use, the total amount was double what was actually needed.

There are significant monetary costs associated with keeping too much inventory. Unfortunately, most nurses are unaware of these costs and continue to engage in overstocking. The major problems arising from too much inventory are discussed below.

All medical supplies cost money and in many cases are expensive. When an excessive inventory is maintained in a nursing unit, the effect is to "tie-up" the monetary value of that excessive amount and deny the use of those funds to the nursing division or hospital for other purposes. For instance, using an example mentioned earlier in the chapter, if a nursing unit maintained a secret and excessive amount (100 items) of 4×3 sponges, costing 90 cents each, the total monetary value of the excess would be $90.00. If the same practices were followed throughout 20 units in a hospital, the total would be $1,800.00

This sum is not available to the nursing division or hospital for other needs (*i.e.*, new equipment purchases, renovation, or investment) and thus represents a major obstacle to profitability. In the simplest case, the money could be invested and earn a rate of interest. However, this potential revenue is lost when excessive inventory "ties-up" funds.

Although no precise estimates of the magnitude of this specific problem are available, it probably represents a significant issue for most nursing units. If this is the case in your unit or hospital, serious attention should be directed at correcting the situation.

A second important problem caused by maintaining too much inventory involves the additional space needed to store it. Excessive supplies often occupy valuable space in patient rooms, unit meeting rooms, or other areas that could be used more efficiently for other purposes. Physical space in any hospital building costs money and should not be used needlessly to accumulate excessive amounts of supplies.

A third problem, while not necessarily caused by excessive inventory, is often closely associated with it in practice. This problem involves the failure to properly rotate dated supplies, resulting in (a) the potential use of outdated or expired products with patients, or (b) monetary losses incurred when outdated supplies are destroyed or discarded. Difficulties with proper stock rotation seem to occur in conjunction with excessive inventory. Extensive stockpiling of supplies tends to foster a careless attitude toward efficient supply use and encourages sloppy rotation of dated items.

Taken together, the aforementioned three problems associated with maintaining too much inventory represent major and unnecessary expenses for many nursing units. Concerted effort is needed to ensure that nurses are aware of these problems, their monetary cost to the unit and institution, and procedures to prevent overstocking.

Effectively addressing the general supply inventory problem in nursing will first require a systematic educational effort to provide nurses with an accurate understanding of (a) the objectives of inventory management, (b) the costs of not enough inventory, (c) the costs of too much inventory, and (d) basic procedures designed to promote efficiency. Without this thorough understanding, success in dealing with the various specific problem areas will be limited.

Several approaches to solving the inventory management problem exist. Some of the more promising strategies are presented in the remainder of this section.

Japanese manufacturers have developed an inventory control system known as Just-In-Time (JIT). Under this system, required materials are delivered by the original supplier to the location where they are used at the precise time that they are needed. For example, in an automobile factory, component parts are delivered by the various suppliers to the location on the assembly line where they are to be used, at the time they are needed.

The advantages of the JIT system are obvious and compelling: (a) supplies are delivered in a timely manner to the point at which they will be used and (b) the manufacturer does not maintain any materials, inventory, thus avoiding any "carrying costs" or storage space problems. Effective functioning of the system requires appropriate and accurate distribution of supplies. If breakdowns occur, the entire production process can be halted — a prospect that is not acceptable in providing patient care.

The concept of JIT inventory control is spreading throughout American business, resulting in unparalleled improvements. Applications within hospital settings in the areas of purchasing and nursing are especially promising. Friesen has proposed a decentralized supply distribution system for use in providing nursing care that contains many of the basic concepts of the JIT approach.[11-13] Friesen argues that supplies should be kept, not in one central location, but rather in specially designed "nurservers," which consist of a pass-through double door cabinet that allows access from both inside and outside a patient's room. Supply technicians are responsible for ensuring that the nurserver is fully stocked daily with basic medical supplies.

This system frees nurses from the task of obtaining necessary supplies and allows them to spend more time in providing direct patient care. Furthermore, required supplies are readily accessible in each patient's room. The Friesen approach has obviously a great deal to recommend it. Shukla reviewed the accumulated research findings evaluating this system and also offered new evidence confirming that significant improvements in time spent in direct patient care and job satisfaction resulted.[10] Although not specifically addressed, reductions in inventory costs also likely occurred.

The Friesen approach is consistent with the philosophy of the JIT concept and facilitates nursing effectiveness while controlling costs. Similar procedures that deliver required supplies in a timely and easily accessible manner, while shifting the burden of inventory maintenance to non-nursing personnel, should meet with success.

The efficiency of the Friesen and other similar systems will increase dramatically as computer terminals in patient rooms become more common. When this occurs, items used can be entered easily into the computer, thus providing an instantaneous record of usage patterns and reorder requirements for central store room personnel.

The specific problem of improper rotation of dated materials should be dealt with by (a) estimating item usage requirements from past data, (b) determining the item's "shelf life" period, (c) communicating with central supply to ensure that usage volume and the shelf life of ordered items are coordinated so that items are used well before their expiration dates, (d) instructing supply personnel to stock from the rear or bottom of a set of items, and (e) instructing nurses to take items from the front or top of a set. Systematic use of these guidelines should correct most stock rotation problems.

The issue of supply storage is a serious one confronting many hospitals and nursing units. Major obstacles exist to effective inventory management and expensive problems are associated with maintaining not enough or too much inventory. Various strategies exist to address these specific areas and should be considered for use in nursing units facing difficulties in inventory management. The ultimate goal is to promote nursing effectiveness and reduce costs. To this end, nurse managers and staff nurses must strive to develop and implement new, innovative, and workable approaches.

CONCLUSIONS

1. The cost of medical supplies used in providing patient care has risen dramatically in recent years, caused mainly by the increasing technological sophistication of medical care and the preference toward disposable, as opposed to reusable, items.

2. Although little precise data exist, substantial anecdotal evidence suggests that the misuse of medical supplies is an extensive and costly problem in nursing.

3. Major potential reasons for the supply misuse problem include (a) a lack of recognition and awareness of the basic issues involved on the part of hospital administrators, nurse managers, and staff nurses, (b) the traditional mode of providing patient care, which generally ignores or deemphasizes efficient supply use, (c) a lack of accurate knowledge concerning actual supply item costs on the part of nursing personnel, (d) a general unfamiliarity with the fundamental principles of efficient use of supplies and the various strategies available, (e) the lack of organizational incentives to encourage cost-effecient use of supplies, (f) a poor nursing attitude towards the entire issue of cost-effectiveness, to include the efficient use of supplies, (g) poor care planning

on the part of staff nurses, and (h) laziness or lack of motivation.

4. A comprehensive corrective program designed to deal explicitly with the supply use problem in nursing includes the following six steps: (a) education and awareness, (b) problem identification, definition, and measurement, (c) participative solution development and goal setting, (d) solution implementation, (e) solution evaluation and revision, and (f) incentives for goal attainment.

5. The first step in promoting more cost-effective use of supplies involves educating nurses regarding the nature and monetary magnitude of the misuse problem and the specific cost of supplies used in the patient care process. This can be accomplished in various ways, including (a) small group discussions, (b) the Price is Right game, (c) posted supply cost lists, or (d) item price stickers.

6. Within each hospital or nursing unit, supply use practices must be carefully reviewed in an effort to identify major problem areas. Once identified and defined, specific problems should be priced to reflect their total cost to the institution. This involves estimating the frequency of the problem and multiplying it by the cost of the item(s) used. Those problems resulting in the highest monetary costs should be addressed first.

7. After supply misuse problems have been prioritized, potential solutions should be participatively developed, soliciting input from all nurses. These efforts should capitalize on the insights, creativity, and ingenuity found in every nurse and encourage the energy created in positive group interaction. In addition, specific target goals for problem reduction should be set in order to motivate and direct nursing behaviors and serve as a yardstick for measuring progress.

8. Once solutions to problems have been identified, the human and material resources necessary to successfully implement a solution must be mobilized by the nurse manager.

9. A critical step in the problem-solving process is to formulate a system to monitor and evaluate the success of a particular solution. Only in this manner is it possible to determine if a strategy is working or not. Potential difficulties can also be identified quickly and corrected. Finally, posting the results of the monitoring process can serve as a powerful motivation function.

10. No program to improve supply use practices is complete without offering incentives to nurses for goal attainment. Ideally, when cost savings are achieved, a percentage of the

total amount should be paid to the nurses involved as a reward and further incentive. This approach is widely and successfully practiced in the private sector and should be implemented in nursing.

11. Major problems exist in the procurement of medical supplies used by nurses in the patient care process including (a) a lack of adequate nursing input into procurement decisions, (b) improper or insufficient product testing, and (c) a lack of standardization in ordering the same item for all units in a hospital. The total monetary cost of these problems can be tremendous. Solutions to the overall supply procurement problem include (a) strong, assertive nursing input into all decisions involving orders for patient care products, (b) the designation of a single nursing administrator to supervise and coordinate all procurement activities, (c) carefully controlled clinical tests of all new products before ordering, (d) the standardization of product orders across all nursing units, and (e) hard bargaining with product manufacturers.

12. An insufficient inventory can lead to (a) misuse of nursing time spent in looking for needed items, (b) possible misuse of substitute products, (c) increased levels of frustration, stress, and dissatisfaction, and (d) potentially life-threatening lapses in care quality. Maintaining too much inventory results in the following problems: (a) hospital funds are "tied-up" in excessive product inventory and not available for other purposes, (b) extra space is required to store the additional inventory, and (c) a commonly related difficulty often arises with improper rotation and use of dated supplies. In correcting these problems, the basic objective is to facilitate nursing effectiveness while minimizing costs. Supply storage and distribution systems that deliver needed materials to nurses in a timely, easily accessible manner and that assign inventory maintenance and control responsibilities to non-nursing personnel are highly recommended.

Questions for Reflection and Discussion

1. How serious do you feel the supply use problem in nursing really is, based on your personal experience and observation?

2. What do you consider the most important causes of the supply use problem in nursing?

3. What are the different ways of educating nurses about the supply use problem and which do you consider are most effective?

4. What are the steps involved in computing costs in a supply use problem and why is this so important?

5. What are the advantages associated with participatively solving nursing unit supply use problems?

6. Why is it important to set specific goals in addressing supply use problems?

7. How would you design an incentive program to encourage nurses to use supplies more cost effectively?

8. What are some of the major problems involved in procuring medical supplies for use in the patient care process?

9. Why should nurses be involved in the supply procurement process and how can they contribute to improved cost-effectiveness in this area?

10. What are the major problems associated with the storage of nursing supply items and how would you recommend that they be dealt with?

REFERENCES

1. Smith TC: Materials management: A model for product review. Nurs Man 16:51–54, 1985
2. Huey FL: Working smart. Am J Nurs 86(6):679–684, 1986
3. Harrell JS, Frauman AC: Prospective payment calls for boosting productivity. Nurs Health Care 6:534–537, 1985
4. Martin DL: Reusing "single use" items: New perspectives. Dimens Health Serv 61:28, 1984
5. Martin DL: Safe reuse of disposables: More conclusive data needed. Dimens Health Serv 62(1):46, 1985
6. Martin DL, Campbell B, Dowler J, Palmer WN: Reuse of disposables—doubts cast on safety and efficacy. Dimens Health Serv 62(8):32–33, 1985
7. Crookston B, Kirchhoff KT: A comprehensive charge system for unit supplies. J Nurs Admin 16:31–34, 1986
8. Madsen NL, Harper RW: Improving the nursing climate for cost containment. J Nurs Admin 15:11–16, 1985
9. Eusebio E, Louisignau K, Horger–Scheuber M, Jorlett J: Product selection in the hospital: Controlling cost. Nurs Man 16:44–46, 1985
10. Shukla RK: Technical and structural support systems and nurse utilization: Systems model. Inquiry 20:381–389, 1983
11. Friesen GA: Integrated communication through construction. Hosp Progr 41 (August):64–67, 1960
12. Friesen GA: A mechanized supply system provides supplies where needed. Hospitals 40 (May):109–112, 1966
13. Friesen GA: Why not build a patient room as a special care unit? Mod Hosp 110 (March):92–93, 1968

9

Improving Patient Scheduling Efficiency

WITH THE introduction and implementation of the diagnostic related group (DRG) system, attention in health care has focused increasingly on the importance of the patient's length of stay (LOS). Hospitals are reimbursed a specific dollar amount for a DRG, based on an average number of days for standard treatment procedures. Costs in excess of the amount are absorbed by the hospital. On the other hand, if an institution can treat and discharge a patient for less than the specified amount, the difference in cost is awarded to the hospital. This system creates strong incentives to efficiently treat patients and discharge them in a timely manner.

The role of nursing in the success of these efforts is critical. The nurse is the primary patient care provider and has responsibility for managing the scheduling of required tests and procedures. Efficiency in patient treatment and scheduling can result in substantial monetary savings, while inefficiency can lead to significant losses.

The primary purpose of this chapter is to introduce the critical path method (CPM) as a tool to improve the scheduling of patients' tests and procedures.

CURRENT SCHEDULING PROBLEMS

Inefficient scheduling of patient tests and procedures is a problem in most hospitals. Prospective payment plans make this a costly problem when the length of stay must be increased in order to accomplish effective treatment. These costs can rise to $500.00 or more for each additional day required. Thus, frequent or chronic scheduling inefficiency can result in significant losses for an institution.

There are multiple causes of patient scheduling problems, which include (1) physicians who fail to discuss and plan treatment procedures with the nurses to allow for appropriate coordination, (2) poor scheduling techniques in the different departments of the hospital (*e.g.*, radiology or the laboratory), (3) inefficient operation of the various departments, resulting in slow patient processing and subsequent backlogs, (4) poor interdepartmental communication, (5) a lack of interdepartmental cooperation, and (6) nursing errors.

Nurses are obviously not the sole cause of scheduling problems, nor can they exert direct control over the physicians and other departments. However, in most institutions, nurses are responsible for managing the scheduling process of patients. Consequently, they must carefully examine their role in eliminating obstacles and promoting efficiency.

There are four major obstacles to efficient scheduling that are under nursing control. The first pertains to improper sequencing of required tests, resulting in an increased LOS. For example, an actual case involved a nurse improperly scheduling a barium enema before an ultrasound of the colon. Since barium interferes with the ultrasound procedure, it was delayed for an additional 24 hours, causing an extra day of hospitalization.

The second nursing obstacle concerns a failure to prepare patients appropriately for required tests or procedures. If, for example, a patient is not placed on NPO prior to a blood test, an additional day may be required to complete the test properly.

A third problem focuses on the lack of nursing assertiveness in dealing with other departments. Given the responsibility of managing the scheduling process, nurses are occasionally not as assertive as they should be in arranging for timely tests and procedures. An actual situation will illustrate this problem. A patient was admitted for DRG 243 (medical back) with a length of stay of 6 days. On the first day, the physician requested a CT scan of the back and the nurse ordered it to be done. The test was not performed until 4 days later and the report was not available in the patient's chart for another 3 days.

On the second day, the electromyogram (EMG) was ordered, but was not performed for 5 days. The patient eventually required 9 days of hospitalization. The total bill was $4,200.00, and the medicare reimbursement was only $2,000.00 for a total loss of $2,200.00 for the hospital.

When the DRG nurse investigated, the assistant head nurse responded that, "we have no control over when the tests are scheduled." Unfortunately, no one in the nursing department had tried to contact the departmental directors involved and or to enlist their cooperation in treating the patient within the 6-day limit. More awareness, responsibility, and assertiveness on the part of the nurses might have prevented this situation from happening. Although the cause of the problem was obviously in the other two departments, the nurse could have attempted to correct the situation.

The fourth and final nursing obstacle to efficient scheduling is a frequent failure to carefully document when and where problems arise. Comprehensive record keeping and documentation can be invaluable in identifying reasons for scheduling delays. For instance, in the aforementioned example, the nurses should have first assertively informed the other two departments involved of the importance of processing the patient within 6 days and requested their cooperation. Then, the time required to actually complete the tests and have them read should have been recorded. In this manner, inefficiencies and delays can be quickly and definitely identified and corrected. If, for example, CT scans of the back routinely take 4 days to complete and another 3 days to be read, this information needs to be made available to the nursing director for discussion at higher levels. Management of the CT scan operation would then hopefully be improved, but at least the nursing department would not be labeled as the cause of the scheduling delay.

In summary, several parties are involved in causing delays in patient scheduling, including physicians, other hospital departments, and the nursing department. These delays can result in significant monetary losses for health care institutions. In most hospitals, the nursing department is charged with the management of the scheduling process. Meeting this responsibility requires that nurses work effectively with physicians and other departments to identify and correct scheduling problems. The critical path method, which is presented in the next section, offers an excellent tool to aid nurses in managing the scheduling process and improving its efficiency.

CRITICAL PATH METHOD

The critical path method (CPM) is a widely used optimal scheduling technique in business and industry. In this section, the fundamental concepts involved in the CPM are introduced, with examples to illustrate its use. (For more detailed information about the procedure, see Lockyer,[1] Martino,[2] or Newbold.[3] It should be pointed out that CPM is similar to other popular scheduling procedures, most notably the program evaluation and review technique (PERT). Given this high degree of similarity, only the CPM is presented.

The CPM was developed originally in 1957 by E.I. DuPont de Nemours and Company, in collaboration with Remington Rand Corporation, to improve the scheduling of factory construction activities and maintenance procedures. Since that time, it has become a popular procedure for monitoring and improving scheduling efficiency. The approach has been used successfully in major construction, manufacturing, and assembly projects. In large scale applications, the CPM is commonly used in conjunction with computers to further enhance its effectiveness.

The primary objective in using the CPM is to identify and define the "critical path" in a particular process. The critical path is defined as the sequence of activities that requires the longest time for completion. Once identified, the critical path will indicate the shortest time necessary to complete a project. If all activities on the critical path are accomplished on time, the overall project will be completed as quickly as possible.

In order to appropriately apply the CPM, the following steps are involved: (1) identify and list all activities needed to complete a particular project, (2) determine the time length associated with each activity, (3) locate and define any sequencing requirements (*i.e.*, activity A before activity B), (4) construct a diagram or flowchart depicting the information in steps 1 to 3, and (5) identify and closely monitor the critical path.

Although the use of the CPM can become complicated in scheduling large projects, the basic concept is simple. Two examples that illustrate this now follow.

The American army has detailed manuals covering all aspects of military operations, which include the preparation of food. Hobson has practical experience in the food service area, having functioned as an enthusiastic member of the kitchen police (KP) in West Germany. Written guidelines pertaining to the preparation of the traditional Thanksgiving dinner are clearcut in specifying the critical path involved. Cooks are instructed to start the fowl first, and then deal with the preparation of the potatoes, vegetables, deserts, and other side dishes. The time required to completely cook the turkey is the critical path in this process and determines the earliest time that the meal can be served.

It was the head cook's responsibility to ensure that the turkeys were started early enough to allow for the noon meal. If this process were delayed by 1 hour, the meal was also delayed by 1 hour. Thus, the importance of closely monitoring the critical path is evident. Activities not on the critical path (*i.e.*, preparation of the other dishes) are not essential for ensuring prompt or timely project completion.

A more commonly used example of the CPM is illustrated in Figure 9-1, which involves a home construction process. The major activities necessary in building a home, from laying the foundation, to framing the house, to painting the interior, are depicted in this figure. The times necessary to complete these activities are also shown. Installation of the plumbing, for example, requires 2 weeks.

The diagram also represents the sequencing relationships between the various activities. For instance, the foundation must be completed before the framing can begin, and the roof must be finished before the exterior can be started. Finally, the diagram shows that some activities can occur simultaneously. In other words, once the framing has been completed, work on the roof, plumbing, and wiring can begin and can continue at the same time.

The critical path in this process is emphasized by the darker

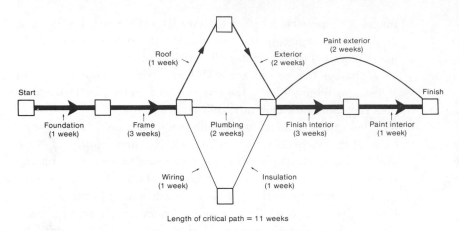

Length of critical path = 11 weeks

FIGURE 9-1. *A common example used to illustrate the usefulness and simplicity of the critical path method is the home building process. The figure provides a flow chart of this process, beginning with laying the foundation, which requires 1 week. The longest sequence of scheduled activities defines the critical path. In this example, the earliest that the house can be completed is 11 weeks.*

lines and arrows. The total time taken is 11 weeks. This critical path represents the sequence of activities that takes the longest time to complete and determines the earliest time that the house could be finished.

Every activity on the critical path must be monitored closely to ensure that the house can be completed in 11 weeks. For example, if the framing activity took 4 weeks, instead of 3 weeks, the house would be finished 1 week later, in 12 weeks. The scheduling and completion of activities off of the critical path are not essential to timely project completion. Therefore, if the wiring activity took 2 weeks instead of 1 week, the house would still be finished in 11 weeks.

Use of the CPM in project scheduling offers several important advantages. Del Mar includes the following: (1) it allows project planning to be developed at any level of detail, (2) it indicates the proper order of activity accomplishment, the degree of task dependency, and scheduling flexibility, (3) the possibility of overlooking tasks that are essential to project completion is drastically diminished, (4) task responsibility and the need for coordination are clarified, (5) accurate time estimates for tasks are conducive to task completion according to schedule, (6) a pictorial plan of action is provided that allows for a broader understanding of responsibilities and interdependence among project participants, (7) potential problem areas can be easily identified and monitored, and (8) a useful framework is provided for making decisions about the costs associated with different project completion times.[4]

These advantages combine to make the CPM a useful and cost-effective scheduling tool.

APPLICATION OF THE CRITICAL PATH METHOD TO PATIENT SCHEDULING

Extensive research and industrial experience have demonstrated that the CPM can be applied effectively in the scheduling of any process involving a set of interrelated activities that must be completed. Within nursing, the potential applications of the CPM are unlimited.[5-7]

Most nurses are implicitly aware of the basic principles underlying the CPM and use them regularly in providing patient care. For instance, when a nurse properly and in a timely manner prepares a patient for an important test, she is attending to essential activities on the patient's critical path to discharge. The nurse is again following the logic of the CPM when a set of required tests is properly sequenced and scheduled.

The purpose of this section is to formally introduce the CPM as a comprehensive conceptual and operational framework for use in patient scheduling. At the conceptual level, every patient has a critical path leading to discharge; in other words, there is some sequence of activities, tests, and procedures that will determine the earliest possible discharge time. This critical path may be complicated, contingent on a host of diagnostic tests, and based on estimates and judgment, but the fact remains that a critical path can be constructed for every patient. For many routine cases, the critical path will be simple and can be standardized easily to improve treatment consistency and efficiency. The challenge to health care providers is to identify and define a patient's critical path as soon as possible and then closely monitor all activities on it to ensure the prompt discharge of patients.

Nursing is typically charged with the responsibility of managing the patient scheduling process. As such, nurses need to take a lead role in coordinating the development of the critical paths of patients. This should be accomplished ideally in conjunction with physicians and other patient service departments involved. Medical and clinical requirements, departmental scheduling constraints, and the need for timely discharge should be discussed openly and should be considered in the formulation of any critical path. Representatives from each of the parties involved should ensure that agreed upon critical path schedules result in high quality patient care and can be followed effectively. By involving physicians and other departments in the development of the critical paths of patients, nurses can hope to identify potential problem areas in advance and correct them before scheduling delays result.

Joint formulation of a critical path for a particular patient is a straightforward process and includes the following steps: (1) list all of the necessary activities, tests, and procedures, with time periods required, (2) identify any sequencing relationships, (3) construct a diagram or flowchart representing the information, and (4) locate the critical path — the sequence of activities, tests, and procedures that requires the longest time to complete.

Two examples are used to illustrate how this process can work and the consequences associated with failing to closely monitor and follow the critical path. A general nursing application of the CPM is presented in Table 9-1. Four tests are necessary (Tests A through D) for this sample case and the required time periods for each are given. Sequencing relationships are also specified in the comments (*i.e.*, Test A must precede Test D). Two optional schedules for this particular situation are given at the foot of Table 9-1. The first one obviously represents an appropriate use of the CPM, resulting in a prompt discharge on the second day. In the second schedule, Test A was not done in the morning of the first day, thus necessitating an additional day of hospitalization.

A more representative and complex example is provided in Figure 9-2. This actual case was originally developed by Hobson and Blaney.[8] It involves an emergency room admission for DRG 177 (uncomplicated peptic ulcer) with an average LOS of 5 days. All of the necessary tests, procedures, and activities are listed in the order that they must be accomplished and interrelationships among them are depicted.

Table 9-1. General Nursing Examples of the Critical Path Method

Sample Case

Tests	Time	Comments
A	5 hrs	Done in laboratory; only in morning; required prior to Test D
B	1 hrs	Done at any time in room
C	1 hrs	Done at any time in room
D	4 hrs	Done in laboratory; only in morning; Test A required first

Optional Schedule 1

	Day 1	Day 2
Morning	A	D
Afternoon	B,C	

Optional Schedule 2

	Day 1	Day 2	Day 3
Morning	B	A	D
Afternoon	C		

The nurse's vital role in performing key functions and managing the overall scheduling process is evident. By closely following this plan, the patient will receive high quality care and will be discharged in 5 days. Failure on the part of the nurse, physician, or other departments to perform required activities in the manner indicated could easily result in extended hospitalization. If, for instance, the nurse fails to properly prepare the patient for required tests, LOS would be extended. Likewise, if delays are encountered in scheduling the required tests, LOS would also be increased.

The advantages of jointly formulating such critical path schedules in cooperation with other hospital departments and physicians are numerous and significant. They include the following: (1) critical paths developed in this manner should be acceptable to all parties involved and should optimally meet medical and scheduling requirements, (2) activities on the critical path can be identified and given special priority and attention, (3) the responsibilities of all parties are delineated, (4) the need for continuing cooperation and communication is emphasized, (5) the causes of scheduling delays can be identified more easily, (6) the consequences of delays are most obvious, and (7) the nurse is provided with a systematic, comprehensive frame-

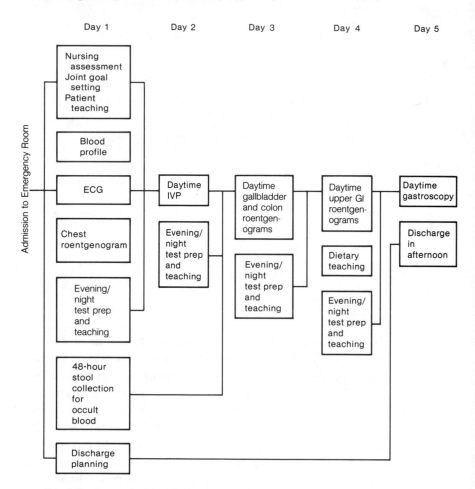

Scheduling the required tests in the proper sequence and appropriately preparing patients for each procedure helps ensure prompt discharge within DRG limits.

FIGURE 9-2. *Applying the CPM to diagnostic tests (for DRG 177, uncomplicated peptic ulcer average length of stay is 5 days). (Hobson CJ, Blaney DR: Techniques that cut costs, not care. Am J Nurs Feb, 1987, pp 185–187)*

work for managing the patient scheduling process in order to provide high quality care as efficiently as possible.

If properly used, the CPM can allow nurses not only to improve the efficiency of the care they provide, but also to improve the entire patient scheduling process, involving other departments and physicians. Success in this effort requires a high degree of communication and cooperation among all parties. Nurses can take a lead role in bringing together other departments and the medical staff to carefully develop the critical paths of patients. Furthermore, for many routine cases, standardized plans could be formulated and used to promote hospital-wide efficiency. Of course, as conditions change, flexibility is needed in order to appropriately modify a patient's critical path. This again necessitates good communication and cooperation.

In the future, central computers will greatly aid this process, allowing nurses to more accurately coordinate patient scheduling requirements with openings in other departments. Ideally, tests, procedures, or activities on a patient's critical path would be given precedence over others. This type of system will greatly improve efficiency throughout a hospital, reduce average LOS, and save a great deal of money.

The CPM can thus best serve nurses in three ways: (1) as a tool to improve efficiency in patient scheduling, (2) as a vehicle to communicate and cooperate with other departments and physicians, and (3) as a framework for recording and documenting scheduling successes and failures. The CPM should be fully integrated with patient care and discharge plans to ensure that total care is delivered in a qualitative and efficient manner. The active cooperation and assistance of other departments and physicians within the hospital is essential to the success of the CPM. Nurses should consequently work to enlist the necessary support from these groups. Finally, the CPM provides a convenient and objective way of locating the causes of scheduling delays. Frequent or chronic problems should be identified and presented to top management for corrective action. Hobson, Blaney, and McHenry have shown that nurses can be successfully trained to use the CPM to significantly reduce patient LOS.[9]

Ideally, nurses need to ensure that they minimize their own scheduling mistakes, assertively set the cooperation of other departments and physicians, and fully document the causes of scheduling delays. Efficiency in patient scheduling should improve significantly by actively using the CPM and following the necessary steps.

SUMMARY AND CONCLUSIONS

1. With the introduction of prospective payment systems in health care, it has become increasingly important to effectively treat patients within the prescribed length of stay.

Additional days of hospitalization can cost an institution as much as $500.00 or more.

2. Problems in the scheduling of patient activities, tests, and procedures are frequently identified as a major cause of unnecessary delays in discharge.

3. Patient scheduling problems are caused by several factors, including: (a) physicians, (b) inefficient operation of patient service departments, (c) poor interdepartmental communication and cooperation, and (d) nursing errors.

4. Nurses are given the responsibility of managing the patient scheduling process in most hospitals.

5. Nursing-based problems that contribute to inefficient patient scheduling include (a) inappropriately sequencing required tests, (b) failure to properly prepare patients, (c) a lack of assertiveness in dealing with other departments in scheduling tests, and (d) insufficient record keeping and documentation concerning causes of scheduling delays.

6. The CPM is a widely used technique in business and industry to improve scheduling efficiency. The primary objective is to identify and define the critical path — the sequence of activities that requires the longest time for completion. Once identified, the critical path should be closely monitored to ensure prompt project completion.

7. Steps involved in applying the CPM include (a) specify and list all activities needed to complete a particular project, (b) determine the length of time associated with each activity, (c) locate and define any sequencing requirements, (d) construct a diagram or flowchart depicting the information collected in steps a to c, and (e) identify and closely monitor the critical path.

8. The CPM can be applied effectively to the problem of patient scheduling. Conceptually, every patient has a critical path to discharge — the sequence of activities, tests, and procedures that takes the longest time to complete and thus determines discharge. The challenge to nursing is to identify and manage a patient's critical path in order to minimize LOS.

9. Patients' critical paths are best developed in cooperation with physicians and other patient service departments. This will ensure that medical and clinical requirements are appropriately addressed, along with departmental scheduling constraints.

10. For many routine cases, simple, standardized critical paths can be developed and used to promote consistency of care and reduce LOS.

11. The advantages of jointly formulating critical paths for patients include (a) the plans that are developed should be acceptable to all parties involved and meet both medical and scheduling requirements, (b) activities on the critical path can be identified and given special priority and attention, (c) the responsibilities of all parties are delineated, (d) the need for continuing cooperation and communication is emphasized, (e) the causes of scheduling delays can be easily located, (f) the consequences of delays are more obvious, and (g) the nurse is provided with a comprehensive framework for managing the patient scheduling process.

12. In order to optimally manage the patient scheduling process, nurses must (a) minimize their own errors and oversights, (b) assertively seek the cooperation of other departments and physicians, and (c) carefully identify and document the causes of delays in order to facilitate their correction.

Questions for Reflection and Discussion

1. Why is the length of stay such an important variable within a prospective payment medical care system?

2. What are the major contributing causes of unnecessary delays in the discharge of patients?

3. Who should manage the patient scheduling process? Give reasons for your answer.

4. What are the principal nursing-based problems that contribute to scheduling delays and which of these is most important in your opinion?

5. What is the critical path method and how has it been used in business and industry? Construct a simple critical path diagram to illustrate how the procedure has been used outside of nursing.

6. Can the CPM realistically be used to improve patient scheduling efficiency? Are there key factors that are essential to the effective use of the CPM?

7. How will staff nurses respond to the CPM?

8. How will other hospital departments and physicians respond to the CPM?

9. What are the major advantages and disadvantages of the CPM for nursing?

10. How could computers enhance the usefulness of the CPM in the scheduling of patients?

11. In addition to patient scheduling, what other areas in nursing could the CPM be successfully applied to?

REFERENCES

1. Lockyer KG: An Introduction to Critical Path Analysis. New York, Pitman Publishing, 1964
2. Martino RL: Critical Path Networks. New York, McGraw–Hill, 1970
3. Newbold P: Principles of Management Science. Englewood Cliffs, NJ, Prentice–Hall, 1986
4. DelMar D: Operations and Industrial Management. New York, McGraw–Hill, 1985
5. Madsen NL, Harper RW: Improving the nursing climate for cost containment. J Nurs Admin 15(3): 11–16, 1985
6. Marriner A: Time management through planning. J Continuing Educ Nurs 14(1): 21–16, 1983
7. Strasen L: Key Business Skills for Nurse Managers. New York, JB Lippincott, 1987
8. Hobson CJ, Blaney DR: Techniques that cut costs, not care. Am J Nurs 87(2): 185–187, 1987
9. Hobson CJ, Blaney DR, McHenry J: Improving the cost effectiveness of nursing practice in a hospital setting. J Continuing Educ Nurs (in press)

Goal Setting as a Potent Motivational Tool for Patients

IN THE health care revolution taking place in the United States, perhaps no single factor is more important and closely scrutinized than patient's length of stay (LOS) in an institution. Recently implemented prospective payment systems reimburse a predetermined amount of money to hospitals, based on an average number of days required to treat a particular principal diagnosis. For those patients covered by prospective payment plans, early discharge leads to higher profits for the hospital, whereas an LOS beyond the prescribed days results in losses. Understandably, LOS has become a critical variable that must be closely monitored and managed.

The patient has a major impact on his own LOS. A key variable is the person's level of motivation to recover. Those individuals with a high level of recovery motivation will generally progress at a more rapid rate, thus reducing LOS. Unfortunately, patients who lack this motivation present nurses with difficult problems and challenges, in addition to significantly hindering their own recovery. Any nurse has probably witnessed countless occasions emphasizing the importance of motivating patients in determining their recovery rate and progress.

Within the hospital setting, the nurse is in a unique position to stimulate the recovery motivation of the patients and facilitate steady progress. A basic component of the nursing process involves formulating conditions to effectively teach patients required recovery and self-care skills, while simultaneously creating a supportive and motivational environment.

The nurse's role in energizing, directing, and sustaining a patient's recovery motivation within the context of goal-setting theory is examined in this chapter. Goal setting offers a simple, yet comprehensive conceptual framework within which to view the patient's motivation process and provides several powerful tools to enhance motivation and learning.

THEORY OF GOAL SETTING

The current theory of goal setting is largely a product of the work of Edwin A. Locke at the University of Maryland. Much of his initial research was conducted in the psychological laboratory using college students and straightforward tasks such as performing numerical calculations. Subsequently, tests of goal-setting theory have also been carried out successfully in various actual organizational sites.

The first comprehensive statement of goal-setting theory was published by Locke in 1968.[1] Although the theory has grown more complicated over the years, the basic hypothesized relationship between goal setting and behavior has remained simple. Locke asserted that the most immediate and important determinant of a person's performance was his work goal or intention (Fig. 10-1); in other words, goals motivate behavior and serve to guide and direct work efforts. Consequently, a person's work goal is generally an excellent indicator of his future performance

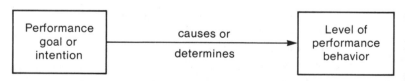

FIGURE 10-1. *Basic mechanism of goal setting.*

level. Locke has argued that this basic concept is fundamental to understanding human motivation, regardless of the theoretical approach taken.[2]

To illustrate how goal-setting theory has been tested, a simple example is taken from among the many studies done in college classrooms. Typically, students are asked at the beginning of a course to state their grade goal; that is, what grade they intend to earn in the class. These stated goals are then compared with final grades and (as you probably suspected) the relationship between the two is strong. Those students expressing goals of "A" or "B" generally did well, whereas students with goals of "C" or "D" usually performed poorly.

Given that goals exert such a powerful influence on subsequent behavior, Locke pointed out that significant improvements in performance could be achieved by systematic goal setting. In order for goal setting to lead to improved performance, however, he emphasized that it was also necessary to provide accurate feedback. Behavioral improvements are contingent on providing information concerning how well or how poorly an individual is doing. Such feedback allows the individual to initiate corrective efforts if desired goals are not being achieved or to continue exhibiting behaviors that have proven successful.

To emphasize the importance of feedback in goal-setting success, imagine setting a grade goal in a college class and then working the entire semester without receiving any performance feedback. Homework grades, test scores, and the instructor's comments would be withheld. Thus, the person would have no idea about how well he was doing. In such situations where feedback is unavailable, goal setting cannot lead to consistent improvements in performance. Therefore, the success of this approach hinges on the provision of accurate and timely feedback about performance.

Locke and other researchers have further refined and developed goal-setting theory since its introduction. Three of the most significant elaborations include (1) the hypothesized superiority of specific *vs* general goals, (2) the hypothesized importance of setting difficult goals, and (3) the hypothesized value of participation in developing work goals.

In the first instance, several theorists have asserted that specific goals will lead to significantly larger improvements in performance than general ones. Specific goals are believed to result in a better focusing of one's attention, motivation, and work effort. Second, it has been hypothesized that relatively difficult goals are superior to easy goals in improving performance. More difficult goals motivate higher levels of effort than easier goals. However, difficult goals must be accepted by the individual as realistic and attainable. An unrealistically difficult goal that cannot be achieved will not be accepted by an individual or serve to guide and direct his performance effort.

Finally, goal-setting theorists have argued that participatively determined work goals are more effective than assigned goals in terms of subsequent acceptance, commitment, and satisfaction. For most people, being allowed the opportunity to participate actively in developing work goals leads to several desirable outcomes. The process of participation increases perceptions of goal ownership, enhances goal acceptance and commitment, and improves overall satisfaction with the goal-setting activity. Participative goal setting is thus generally considered superior to assigned or autocratic goal setting.

RESEARCH RESULTS

Since its introduction in the mid-1960s, goal-setting theory has stimulated a large volume of research and is the focus of a great deal of continuing attention.[3] Periodic reviews of this literature are consistent in their finding that goal setting is effective in improving performance.[3-5] For example, Locke and associates reviewed goal-setting studies from 1969 to 1980.[5] Of the 110 published articles, 99 of them found that goal setting resulted in improved performance, or a success percentage in excess of 90%. The researchers concluded that the "beneficial effect of goal setting on task performance is one of the most robust and replicable findings in the psychological literature" (p 145).[5] The fact that goal setting has been found to work equally well in laboratory or field environments is particularly important.

Locke and associates asserted that goal setting affects performance in any one of four ways: (1) by directing one's attention and action, (2) by mobilizing an individual's effort, (3) by sustaining effort over time, and (4) by motivating the person to formulate strategies for goal attainment.[5]

The magnitude of improvement in task performance brought about by goal setting has been estimated by Locke, Feren, McCaleb, Shaw, and Denny.[6] They reviewed the available experimental field studies involving goal setting used in actual organizations. The median improvement in performance as a function of goal setting was 16%. When goal setting was combined with monetary incentives, the median improvement in performance rose to 40%. Thus, goal setting has consistently demonstrated a substantial impact on performance, especially when combined with monetary rewards.

The potential improvements in performance and productivity can result in significant monetary savings for organizations. Latham and Baldes examined the use of goal setting with truck drivers hauling logs in the timber industry.[7] Over 9 months, the dramatic increase in timber tonnage transported saved the company over $250,000.00. This example and other similar studies suggest that goal setting can have an important effect on profits.

Although the major conclusion in the goal-setting literature is that the technique consistently improves the performance, researchers have also addressed several other related issues. These include (1) the role of performance feedback in goal setting, (2) the relative effectiveness of specific *vs* general goals, (3) the merits of setting hard, acceptable goals as opposed to easy ones, (4) the value of participation in the goal-setting process, and (5) the impact of supportiveness in facilitating goal setting.

Research results are conclusive regarding the necessity of performance feedback in the goal-setting process. Without accurate, systematic information about performance behavior, goal setting alone does not result in improvement. Individuals need feedback in order to maintain appropriate levels of performance or initiate corrective action when deficiencies are detected. Thus, adequate performance feedback is necessary for the effectiveness of goal setting.

Research findings are equally conclusive in demonstrating that specific goals are superior to general goals, such as "do our best" or "try hard." Individuals with specific goals are better able to direct and focus their work efforts and monitor their progress. General goals provide only an ambiguous objective and no clearcut yardstick to evaluate achievement. Consequently, specificity is always recommended when setting goals.

Several studies have addressed the relative impact of hard goals *vs* easy ones. Findings suggest that hard goals lead to higher levels of performance than easy goals, but only when the hard goals are fully accepted. In other words, setting hard goals that are perceived as unacceptable and unattainable by individuals will have little impact on their performance. Hard goals, if accepted as legitimate and attainable, function to stimulate performance over and above what is observed when easy goals are used. Therefore, when using goal setting, a concerted effort should be made to employ goals that are difficult and challenging, but not so difficult as to be viewed as unrealistic.

A great deal of research has been done on the efficacy of participatively determined, as compared to assigned, goals. Participation entails the active involvement of the individuals who are using the goal-setting technique in the formulation of what their goals should be. The use of assigned goals involves providing task goals to individuals without prior consultation or discussion.

Findings from this research indicate that there are not consistent differences in the performance level between participative and assigned goals.[8] The act of goal setting alone, whether done in a participative or assigned manner, appears to serve to increase performance. The use of participative approaches, however, does offer several valuable advantages that indirectly influence performance.

First, the use of participation serves to reduce resistance to plans, changes, or goals. By participating in the planning or goal-setting process, an individual develops feelings of ownership and is thus less likely to resist the plans or goals that are decided on. Second, in a similar sense, the acceptance of and commitment to goals that are participatively determined tend to be higher than with assigned goals. The notion of perceived ownership again plays an important role in stimulating goals acceptance and commitment. Finally, for most people, participation in goal setting leads to enhanced levels of satisfaction with the overall process; in other words, being given an opportunity for genuine input typically leads to feelings of satisfaction with the overall goal-setting process.

People do not generally like to be told precisely and completely what their work goals will be. Participation is thus recommended as a useful means of improving the impact of goal setting.

Locke and associates briefly discuss the emerging research on the concept of supportiveness in goal setting.[5] Latham and Saari initially introduced the notion and defined it as including friendliness, listening to a person's opinions about his goals, and encouraging questions, and asking rather than telling people what to do.[9] Although there have been limited research tests of the impact of supportiveness, Locke and associates asserted that it may be even more important than participation in facilitating the effectiveness of goal setting.[5] They concluded by requesting more research on this promising concept. Theoretically, the potential value and use of supportiveness are compelling, and thus, future research is expected to confirm its significance.

The extensive literature on goal setting thus confirms the efficacy of the technique in effecting improvements in task performance. Although this research has been conducted primarily in either laboratory or industrial settings, the findings have important implications for nurses regarding the motivation of patients.

APPLICATIONS OF GOAL SETTING THEORY AND RESEARCH TO NURSING PRACTICE

The importance of motivating patients as a primary determinant of the recovery rate has been emphasized. The patient should be viewed ideally as an integral member of the health care team and his active participation and cooperation are essential to the ultimate success and efficiency of the care process.

Unfortunately, as several authors have pointed out,[10,11] the patient is often excluded from involvement in the process of developing and implementing care goals and plans. Alexy noted that "the patient has been a passive recipient of care, not allowed the responsibility for even limited aspects of the care plan until the moment of discharge" (p 298).[10]

The success of nursing care in general and goal setting in particular clearly depends on the active inclusion of patients in the formulation and implementation of care goals and plans. Bandman and Bandman have argued that nurses have an ethical responsibility to involve patients in the development of individualized goals and plans for their care.[12] For the purposes of this chapter, without active patient involvement and cooperation, goal setting cannot be effective in motivating recovery and reducing LOS.

Goal setting is not a new concept in nursing. It is an important component in the basic nursing process. However, given the accumulation of new research findings on the effectiveness of goal setting in increasing performance, several potentially significant nursing applications are possible. The focus in this section is on the use of goal setting in motivating a patient's recovery.

With this in mind, recall that Locke and associates[5] concluded that goal setting affects performance in any one of four ways: (1) by directing one's attention and action, (2) by mobilizing an individual's efforts, (3) by sustaining effort over time, and (4) by motivating the person to formulate strategies for goal attainment. Within nursing, these mechanisms hold tremendous potential for improving the overall patient care process, increasing patient recovery motivation, and reducing LOS. The challenge for nurses involves understanding, mastering, and applying goal-setting techniques to achieve these objectives.

In this section, practical applications of the goal setting research are presented, along with a format for implementing these strategies. Three specific areas are addressed: (1) the formulation and clarification of end goals that must be met prior to discharge, (2) the determination of daily subgoals, and (3) the nurse's role as a source of feedback, support, and encouragement.

Progressive nurses in the United States have already successfully applied many of the lessons learned from the goal-setting literature. When appropriate, these published examples are cited to illustrate how goal setting can be used in practice.

Formulation and Clarification of End Goals

In order for goal setting to be effective in motivating a patient's recovery and in decreasing LOS, a necessary first step involves the unambiguous specification of end goals that must be met prior to discharge; in other words, what specific conditions, skills, or abilities must be achieved before a patient can be released from the hospital. These end goals should be developed and shared with the patient as soon as possible to enable the person to actively work together with the nurse toward a timely discharge. If end goals are not explicitly provided for a patient, an outstanding opportunity to mobilize and direct the patient's effort and attention toward goal attainment is lost.

A convenient format for use in the goal-setting process is provided in Figure 10-2. The specification of both explicit end goals and daily subgoals are included in Figure 10-2. A written goal-setting plan in this basic format should be developed and actively used with each patient in order to structure and facilitate a timely recovery.

Unfortunately, as Alexy,[10] Giloth,[11] and others have observed, the patient is often excluded from the process of specifying care goals and developing the care plan. This can result in many undesirable consequences. Perhaps a personal example can illustrate the frustration and inefficiency that can arise when patients are not informed and involved in the care process.

In the early 1980s, Hobson entered the hospital in late December for a scheduled tonsillectomy. Upon admission, he was told that the length of stay for adults varied from 2 to 4 days, depending on a nebulous set of criteria that would be explained fully after surgery by the nurse.

The holiday season provided ample motivation to get out of the hospital as quickly as possible. Thus, soon after surgery, the attending staff nurse was asked (in writing) to describe the criteria used in making discharge decisions; in other words, what "tricks" needed to be performed in order for a patient to be discharged in 2 days as opposed to 4 days. She was uncertain as to exactly what the decision was based on and summoned the head nurse. She, in turn, responded that several factors were important, such as, body temperature, bleeding, fluid intake, eating habits, and how soon the patient could walk unassisted.

More specific information on these criteria was requested from the head nurse; such as, what the temperature needed to be, how much fluid needed to be consumed, how much and what types of food needed to be eaten, and how long a patient should be able to work unassisted. Unfortunately, she was unable to answer these questions. The physician, who was also of little help, said that it all depended on the circumstances.

The frustration that this experience caused was considerable. The decision to discharge the patient in this and other routine cases was obviously based on levels attained on some set of

Subgoals — End Goals

Day 1 Specific Goals	Day 2 Specific Goals	Day 3 Specific Goals	Day 4 Specific Goals	Prior to Discharge the Patient Must be Able to:
(1) _____	(1) _____	(1) _____	(1) _____	(1) _____
(2) _____	(2) _____	(2) _____	(2) _____	(2) _____
(3) _____	(3) _____	(3) _____	(3) _____	(3) _____
(4) _____	(4) _____	(4) _____	(4) _____	(4) _____
(5) _____	(5) _____	(5) _____	(5) _____	(5) _____

FIGURE 10-2. Goal setting and patient care focus.

criteria. Regrettably, these "magic numbers" were not delineated and agreed on to the extent that they could be communicated clearly to the patient. Thus, in this instance, the patient had a tremendous level of motivation to recover and leave the hospital, but was hindered in this effort by the lack of clear-cut end goals guiding the care plan and serving as the basis for the discharge decision.

Hospitals can no longer afford to miss opportunities to enlist the active participation and cooperation of patients in the care process. Nurses must take a lead role in this effort, which should begin with the specification of end goals to be achieved prior to discharge.

Ideally, building on the research results in goal setting, end goals should be as specific as possible and they should be participatively determined. General goals do not work as well as more specific ones. For example, Rice and Johnson found that specific preadmission self-instructional material (*i.e.*, explicit goal information) as compared to general material resulted in more complete and efficient learning of exercise behaviors for a group of 130 surgical patients.[13] Specificity is thus highly desirable when formulating end goals.

Participation in the determination of personal health goals was examined by Hefferin,[14] using two groups of patients in a veterans' hospital. One group participated in the development of their goals, while the second group received goals developed by nurses. Hefferin found that the participative group achieved more goals within a shorter time than the assigned goal group. In another study addressing the effects of participation, Alexy found no differences in goal attainment between participative and assigned goal groups of patients involved in a health risk reduction project.[10] Unfortunately, goal specificity and difficulty were not controlled in this study, nor were goal acceptance, commitment, or overall patient satisfaction measured. Participative approaches have not been found to result in improved performance compared to the use of assigned goals. However, differences are found on such variables as goal acceptance and commitment and general satisfaction with the goal-setting process.

Consequently, the limited available nursing research bearing on the merits of participation in goal setting, when combined with the more extensive industrial literature, strongly suggests that patients should participate in developing end goals for their own treatment. Perceived ownership of end goals should significantly enhance acceptance, commitment, and satisfaction with the process.

End goals should be established as soon as possible in order to facilitate active patient/nurse cooperation. With many scheduled surgical procedures, this increasingly means setting these goals prior to admission. Rice and Johnson noted that preoperative teaching of surgical patients about activities that they will be required to perform after surgery is recommended in leading nursing textbooks and is practiced in many hospitals in the United States.[13] Numerous writers have argued cogently for the value of comprehensive preadmission processing of surgical patients to include systematic teaching and goal setting.[11,15,16]

The time prior to admission offers an excellent opportunity to begin the goal-setting process by identifying end goals that must be achieved prior to discharge and beginning efforts to attain them. As Rice and Johnson indicated,[13] patients have more time available for learning and practice prior to entering the hospital and are typically less anxious. Clarifying recovery expectations before admission can help the patient begin to prepare mentally, emotionally, and physically for the scheduled surgery and a speedy recovery.

Tests of these types of programs have generally shown them to be successful. For example, Fortin and Kirouac compared one group of preoperative patients that received preadmission instruction on required postsurgical exercises with a second control group that received no instruction at all.[17] Findings indicated that the patients with preadmission instructions had higher physical function scores, requested less pain medication, and had higher reported levels of physical comfort during the postoperative period, as compared to the control group. Giloth reported that several hospitals have developed preadmission training programs for patients with arthroplasty, focusing on the skills and exercises required after surgery.[11] These programs have resulted in significant decreases in average LOS. Finally, in the study mentioned earlier by Rice and Johnson,[13] the use of preadmission self-instruction booklets was found to result in substantial reductions in the nursing time spent in teaching postoperative exercises to 130 surgical patients.

The accumulated research evidence demonstrates convincingly that the initiation of the goal-setting process, to include the identification of end goals, can be accomplished effectively for surgical patients prior to their admission and often results in a shorter LOS. The use of preadmission goal setting and instruction should be examined thoroughly and the approach should be used whenever possible.

With other patients, when preadmission consultation is not possible, end goals required prior to discharge should be developed and shared by them at the earliest possible time. This will allow the patient to work more effectively with the nurse toward a timely discharge.

The goal-setting process thus begins with the formulation of end goals that must be met prior to discharge. End goals should ideally be as specific as possible and should be developed in cooperation with the patient. They should also be identified as soon as possible in the patient care process to allow the patient to accurately direct his efforts toward goal attainment and discharge. Research has shown that in many routine surgical cases, the specification of end goals can be completed prior to admission.

Determination of Daily Subgoals

Once end goals for a particular patient have been established, the next step in the goal-setting process involves working backwards to determine the specific daily subgoals that must be accomplished in order to achieve the end goals, so that the patient is discharged in a timely manner. Locke and associates recognized the conceptual importance of sub- or intermediate goals in the overall effectiveness of the goal-setting process and deplored the lack of research on this topic.[5] Clearly, in order for goal setting to work, the manner in which end goals can be achieved must be well defined. Most end goals cannot be met with one step, but rather involve a series of small steps, leading to the desired outcome.

For example, with newly diagnosed diabetics, one important end goal involves the self-administration of insulin. Competence in this critical task is not acquired in a single step or attempt. Instead, instruction and practice are necessary to fully master the skill.

A helpful format for conceptualizing the overall goal-setting process, consisting of well-defined end goals and a set of daily subgoals, is provided in Figure 10-2. Subgoals should have the following characteristics: (1) specificity, (2) participative development, and (3) challenge. A central theme of this chapter has been the value of goal specificity. In order for goal setting to work effectively in motivating a patient's recovery, daily subgoals must be as specific as possible. They should also be formulated in a participative manner with the patient. By encouraging participation and cooperation, the nurse can significantly increase goal acceptance and commitment, as well as satisfaction with the process itself.

Finally, daily subgoals should be as challenging as possible. Difficult goals, if accepted, are superior to easy goals in stimulating performance. The key variable, however, concerns goal acceptance. Difficult goals must be accepted as attainable and realistic by the patient in order for them to facilitate performance improvement. This is one reason why participation in goal setting is so highly recommended, especially when setting difficult goals.

The nurse should work with the patient to establish daily subgoals that are genuinely challenging, without being overwhelming. Of course, the nurse must be sensitive to individual differences in patients and she must realize that, in many cases, the best advice is to start slowly and build momentum and confidence through a series of successes. Thus, for many patients, relatively easy initial subgoals will allow them to experience success in goal attainment and thereby foster increased motivation and confidence. As easy goals are attained, subsequent subgoals can be formulated that are increasingly more difficult.

Steady patient progress and confidence are critical variables in this process. Thus, the nurse must use good judgment, based on clinical training and experience, to determine the optimal amount of challenge appropriate for a particular patient.

Every attempt should be made to minimize errors involved in developing goals that are too difficult for the patient. The resultant experience of failure can serve to significantly hamper their recovery and impair their confidence and motivation. Again, the best advice is to start slowly, to build on successes, and to gradually increase the difficulty level of goals as the patient demonstrates the ability to handle them.

Two important points about daily subgoals must be made. First, revisions should be initiated in the goal-setting plan as soon as conditions change substantially. The goal-setting plan of including the daily subgoals is not rigid. For example, if a patient makes extraordinary progress and easily attains all of the subgoals for a particular day, the patient and nurse should not be prevented from moving to the subgoals listed for the following day. Such progress should be encouraged and can be intentionally built into the goal-setting plan as a motivational technique.

For most patients, it would be a tremendous confidence booster to easily complete all of the designated subgoals on the first day and then to progress to those for the next day. Nurses should be aware of these powerful motivational aspects of goal setting and should use them in the care process.

Just as daily subgoals can be revised upward to include goals for the following day, a patient's difficulties or failures should result in similar downward modifications. Experiences of failure for patients are not conducive to good mental and emotional health, or rapid recovery. Consequently, revisions should be made quickly once a patient experiences major problems in attaining a particular goal.

A second important point about daily subgoals concerns the need for more research to address the relative effectiveness of different care plans or subgoal sequences in promoting a patient's recovery. There is often little uniformity or standardization in care plans or subgoal sequences or even a routine. The approach taken depends on the individual nurse involved.

Although it is desirable to personalize care plans to meet the unique needs of patients, research can be useful in identifying (1) standardized care plans or subgoal sequences that work most effectively and (2) important individual difference variables that should be taken into account when formulating a plan for a particular patient.

This general issue was first brought to our attention as a result of a goal-setting exercise used in nursing seminars conducted in hospitals in the United States. In the exercise, nurses were asked to use a form, similar to the one provided in Figure 10-2, to develop a set of daily subgoals for a patient, described as a 65-year-old, newly diagnosed diabetic. For the sake of simplicity, explicit end goals were listed as (1) the self-administration of insulin, and (2) the selection of an appropriate diet. Participants were then asked to work backwards and develop a set of daily subgoals that would result in the attainment of the two stated end goals in an appropriate, efficient, and effective manner.

The responses generated with respect to the first end goal — the self-administration of insulin — were particularly interesting. Nurses recognized uniformly that a common set of subtasks needed to be completed in order to achieve competence. These included (1) basic verbal instruction concerning the purpose of insulin, the function of syringes, and the techniques involved in self-administration, (2) a demonstration by a nurse of drawing-up insulin, (3) practice by a patient in drawing up insulin, (4) observation of the nurse administering insulin to the patient, (5) practice using the syringe, and finally (6) practice in actual self-administration.

At this point, the commonality in nursing responses ended. Tremendous disparity was found in both the length of stay required to achieve the stated goals and the specific sequencing of subgoals best suited for the situation. For example, LOS varied from zero to 4 days, with some nurses asserting that the patient should be discharged immediately from the hospital and treated on an out-patient basis, whereas others insisted that effective teaching and treatment could only be accomplished in 4 full days of hospitalization.

The differences in subgoal sequencing were also substantial. For instance, most nurses saved the task of actual self-administration until the third or fourth day, after a great deal of instruction and practice. On the other hand, some nurses scheduled actual self-administration for the first day, followed by in-depth instruction and practice. The rationale for this second approach was that the patient is typically so tense and anxious about the inevitable use of the syringe that it is best to "get it over with quickly and early" so that the person can then relax and better concentrate on learning more about the disease and its treatment. Some preliminary research supports the effectiveness of this strategy.[18]

The key point is that there is substantial variation in the way nurses approach the treatment of diabetes, both in terms of a patient's length of stay in hospital and subgoal sequencing. Similar variation would probably also be found with other disease categories. What is sorely needed is systematic clinical research to evaluate the relative effectiveness of different care plans and subgoal sequences in order to identify those that work best for the patient, nurse, and hospital. Once identified, these proven approaches could then be used with all routine cases. Nursing judgment would be required to initiate changes in the standard approach to accommodate the unique needs of a particular patient.

In conclusion, once end goals have been established, it is then necessary to formulate a set of daily subgoals that will result in a timely recovery and discharge. These subgoals should be as specific as possible, participatively developed, and challenging, though not overwhelming. The set of daily subgoals serves as a road map and plan for a patient's recovery and functions to motivate and direct behaviors toward discharge. Established subgoal sequences should be revised when necessary for an individual patient and more research is needed to rigorously evaluate the differential effectiveness of various approaches.

Nurse as A Source of Feedback, Support, and Encouragement

Within the patient care context, the effectiveness of goal setting depends on the active involvement of the nurse in developing, implementing, and monitoring goal-setting plans. In order for this process to be successful in promoting a patient's recovery, the nurse must also perform a vital function as a source of feedback, support, and encouragement.

The importance of feedback in goal setting has been conclusively established. Without information concerning the level, quality, or effectiveness of performance, improvements as a result of goal setting alone are not possible. People need feedback information in order to determine how well they are doing. If they are making progress or performing well, feedback serves to identify problem areas in need of correction.

The requirement for adequate feedback in patient teaching has been recognized by writers and researchers in nursing.[13,19] The nurse must ideally assume responsibility for ensuring that timely and accurate feedback is available to patients throughout the teaching and goal-setting process. Patients need information about how well they are doing and goal progress if the process is to function appropriately.

The nurse represents perhaps the single most important

source of feedback information available to patients concerning the "correctness" or adequacy of their goal-directed behaviors. From the patient's perspective, the nurse is the expert, by virtue of her clinical training and experience, on care goals and how to best achieve them. The nurse is also regularly in contact with the patient and has ample opportunity to provide relevant feedback about performance.

However, although it is the responsibility of the nurse to ensure that a patient has access to feedback information, it is not necessary or advisable for the nurse to function as the sole source of that information. Instead, nurses should teach patients how to evaluate the correctness or adequacy of their own behaviors. This is especially important when using written preadmission teaching and goal-setting plans. For example, Rice and Johnson,[13] recognizing the critical value of self-monitoring and feedback, provided written preadmission exercise instructions to a group of surgical patients which contained explicit standards to evaluate the adequacy of specific procedures. Thus, in teaching a deep-breathing exercise, one of the steps was "Hold your breath for 2 to 3 seconds. Count to yourself 1-2-3. Your abdomen should not move."

In this seemingly simple step, the researchers have provided information on (1) how to hold your breath for 2 to 3 seconds — "Count to yourself 1-2-3," and (2) how to determine if you are doing this correctly — "your abdomen should not move." This type of information allows the patient, not only to perform the exercise better, but also to assess effectiveness.

Whenever possible, nurses need to explicitly teach patients how to monitor their own progress and measure it against daily subgoals and end goals. Another simple example might be helpful. If a particular patient has a daily subgoal that involves the consumption and discharge of a certain volume of fluid, goal progress can be self-monitored by using a urine collection container and by explaining to the patient how to use, read, and interpret it. Thus, as the patient drinks and discharges fluid, he can immediately obtain feedback information concerning progress towards the goal for that day.

Although teaching patients self-monitoring skills is advisable, nurses should nevertheless periodically provide personal feedback to the patient concerning goal progress. This serves three basic functions: (1) to verify the accuracy of the patient's self-feedback, (2) to discern potential problems in the patient's self-monitoring techniques, and (3) to further motivate the patient by showing personal concern and interest.

Up to this point, feedback has been considered primarily in terms of its informational value; that is, providing the patient with necessary data concerning the adequacy, level, or quality of his behavior. Such informational feedback is essential for the effectiveness of the goal-setting process.

Feedback can also be considered in terms of its evaluative function. In contrast to strictly informational feedback, evaluative feedback consists of a subjective assessment of how well or how poorly a patient is performing.

To illustrate the difference between the two, consider the following examples of each one: "Your urine collection container has 23 fluid ounces in it" *vs* "You are doing a great job drinking more fluids today." In the first case, the feedback provides descriptive information only, whereas in the second example, the feedback is of an evaluative nature.

Positive evaluative feedback serves as a powerful incentive for most people and significantly increases the levels of motivation. Informational feedback can also increase motivation, but evaluative comments are more effective in encouraging people to try harder and do better.

The nurse is in a unique position to provide evaluative feedback to patients concerning goal progress. The impact of such positive evaluative feedback is dramatic and can be readily observed with most patients. Consequently, nurses should recognize this and appreciate the powerful impact that they can have on the motivation of patients and on goal progress through the use of evaluative feedback. Time spent in praising a patient's performance will reap several benefits: (1) the patient will feel better about himself, (2) the patient will be more motivated to continue working hard to attain care goals, and (3) the nurse will feel better as a consequence of having given the positive feedback to another human being.

People like to think of themselves as winners. When this occurs, people feel better about themselves and life in general. Nurses can take advantage of this invaluable information and use it in the goal-setting process. As mentioned earlier, initial daily subgoals can be set that are relatively easy to attain. When the patient accomplishes these goals, the nurse should supply well deserved positive feedback. The goal attainment success experience, combined with the positive feedback from the nurse, can be counted on to make the patient feel like a winner, thereby feeling better about himself and typically increasing his desire to work harder towards continued goal attainment. Thus, the best advice to nurses is not to underestimate the powerful effect that positive feedback can have on a patient's well-being and rate of recovery.

The patient who tries and fails to attain daily subgoals requires special attention from the nurse. Experiences of failure are not conducive to a patient's mental and emotional health or recovery. Consequently, if a patient is experiencing major difficulties in attaining a specific goal, the nurse should act to revise the goal in a downward direction, while at the same time reinforcing the person for trying to succeed. In such situations, the nurse must provide positive feedback to the patient for his efforts. No one feels good about failing, but reassurance that one's efforts are recognized helps to ease the pain. Therefore, patients should be rewarded verbally, not only for attaining their goals, but also for trying hard to attain them.

Unfortunately, some patients refuse to try at all. In these cases, goal setting will not work and the nurse must rely on her counseling skills or the assistance of mental health professionals to explore the reasons why the patient fails to even try to attain treatment goals.

The importance of the nurse's support and encouragement in the success of goal setting in the patient care process is obvious and recognized. The provision of psychological support to patients is a widely accepted integral part of professional nursing practice.[20-22]

Unfortunately, Devine and Cook cited evidence indicating that psychological support levels in actual nursing practice were often disappointingly low.[23-25] The researchers called for increased attention to this essential nursing function and supported their argument with the results of a meta-analytic review of 49 studies addressing the impact of psychoeducational interventions on postsurgical LOS. Psychoeducational interventions were defined in terms of three components: (1) information concerning surgical procedures and recovery, (2) specific skills training, and (3) psychological support.

Devine and Cook found that such treatment combinations resulted in an average reduction in postsurgical LOS of 1.31 days.[23] The potential monetary savings to a health care institution are obvious and substantial. The researchers asserted that well-formulated psychoeducational interventions constitute an excellent means of enhancing a patient's recovery, that they improve the level of a patient's satisfaction and well-being, and that they also increase the job satisfaction of the nurses involved.

However, successful interventions require considerable nursing time and effort. If nurses are expected to provide this type of intensive, high quality care, additional staffing demands will arise. Given the documented, bottom-line impact of psychoeducational interventions on LOS, hiring the additional nursing personnel required may constitute a cost-effective strategy.

The nurse therefore plays an essential role in the goal-setting process as a source of feedback, support, and encouragement. By systematically providing both informational and evaluative feedback, the nurse can significantly increase a patient's motivation for recovery and can thereby decrease LOS.

CONCLUSIONS

1. Given the introduction of prospective payment systems, a patient's length of stay has become a major focus of efforts to control costs in hospitals.

2. A patient's level of motivation is a major determinant of his rate of recovery and thus his LOS.

3. The nurse is in a unique position to exert a powerful influence on a patient's motivation to recover. Goal-setting theory provides a comprehensive conceptual framework for evaluating and enhancing a nurse's ability to stimulate a patient's motivation.

4. Goal-setting theory posits that the most important determinant of a person's level of performance is his work goal or intention. The role of timely, accurate feedback in this process is critical.

5. Extensions of the basic theory of goal setting include (a) the hypothesized superiority of specific *vs* general goals, (b) the hypothesized value of setting difficult goals, if they are ac-

cepted as attainable, and (c) the hypothesized role of participation in increasing the effectiveness of goal setting.

6. Research findings indicate that in over 90% of the studies that have been conducted, goal setting has resulted in significant increases in task performance. The median performance improvement in actual organizations has been 16%. When combined with monetary incentives, the median improvement rises to 40%.

7. Additional conclusions derived from the goal-setting research include (a) accurate, timely performance feedback is essential to the effectiveness of goal setting, (b) specific goals are superior to general goals in stimulating performance, (c) difficult goals, if accepted, lead to higher performance levels than easy goals, (d) the use of participation in the goal-setting process results in less resistance to change, improved goal acceptance and commitment, and higher overall satisfaction, and (e) supportiveness in goal setting plays an important role in facilitating the entire process.

8. The goal-setting research can be applied to the issue of motivating a patient's recovery in three major areas: (a) the formulation and clarification of end goals that must be met prior to discharge, (b) the participative determination of challenging, specific daily subgoals, and (c) the nurse as a source of feedback, support, and encouragement.

9. Additional, carefully designed and controlled nursing research is needed in order to identify optimal care plans and daily subgoal sequences that result in efficient patient care and timely discharge.

Questions for Reflection and Discussion

1. Why is patient LOS so important in containing rising health costs?

2. What is a patient's motivation and how is it related to LOS?

3. How can the nurse influence a patient's motivation to recover? Give examples to illustrate your answer.

4. What is the basic premise of goal setting, and why is it so useful in understanding human behavior?

5. Explain the role of performance feedback in the goal-setting process.

6. Why should specific goals be superior to general goals?

7. Why is acceptance so critical when setting difficult goals?

8. What impact do you feel participation has on the goal-setting process? Give examples to illustrate your answer.

9. Briefly summarize the major findings in the goal-setting literature.

10. Why are end goals so important in motivating timely patient discharge?

11. What important considerations should the nurse keep in mind when developing daily subgoals for a patient?

12. How important is the nurse's role in the goal-setting process as a source of performance feedback, support, and encouragement?

13. How would you design a study to evaluate the relative effectiveness of different care plans or subgoal sequences in facilitating the timely discharge of patients?

REFERENCES

1. Locke EA: Toward a theory of task motivation and incentives. Organizational Behavior and Human Performance 3: 157–189, 1968
2. Locke EA: The ubiquity of technique of goal setting in theories of approaches to employee motivation. Acad Man Rev 3: 594–601, 1978
3. Schneider B: Organizational behavior. In Rosenzweig MR, Porter LW (eds): Annual Review of Psychology, Vol 35. Palo Alto, CA, Annual Reviews, 1985
4. Latham GP, Yukl GA: A review of research on the application of goal setting in organizations. Acad Man J 18: 824–845, 1975
5. Locke EA, Shaw KN, Saari LM, Latham GP: Goal setting and task performance: 1969–1980. Psychol Bull 90: 125–152, 1981
6. Locke EA, Feren DB, McCaleb VM et al: The relative effectiveness of four methods of motivating employee performance. In Duncan K, Gruenberg M, Wallis D (eds): Changes in Working Life. New York, Wiley, 1980
7. Latham GP, Baldes JJ: The "practical significance" of Locke's theory of goal setting. J Appl Psychol 60: 122–124, 1975
8. Locke EA, Schweiger DM: Participation in decision-making: One more look. In Staw BM (ed): Research in Organizational Behavior, Vol 1. Greenwich, CT, JAI Press, 1979
9. Latham GP, Saari LM: Importance of supportive relationships in goal setting. J Appl Psychol 64: 151–156, 1979
10. Alexy B: Goal setting and health risk reduction. Nurs Res 34: 283–288, 1985
11. Giloth B: Incentives for planned patient education. QRB 11: 295–300, 1985
12. Bandman EL, Bandman B: Nursing Ethics in the Life Span. Norwalk, CT, Appleton–Century–Crofts, 1985
13. Rice VH, Johnson JE: Preadmission self-instruction booklets, postadmission exercise performance, and teaching time. Nurs Res 33: 147–151, 1984

14. Hefferin EA: Health goal setting: Patient–nurse collaboration at Veterans Administration facilities. Milit Med 144(12): 814–822, 1979
15. Granatir T: Peer review organizations: Implications for discharge planning. Discharge Planning Update 5: 4–10, 1985
16. Smeltzer CH, Flores SM: Preadmission discharge planning: Organization of a concept. J Nurs Admin 16: 18–24, 1986
17. Fortin F, Kirouac S: A randomized controlled trial of preoperative patient education. Int J Nurs Stud 7: 173–184, 1976
18. Blevins D, Cassmeyer V: The patient with diabetes mellitus. In Long B, Phipps W (eds): Essentials of Medical-Surgical Nursing. St. Louis, CV Mosby, 1985
19. Redman BK: The Process of Teaching in Nursing, 3rd ed. St. Louis, CV Mosby, 1976
20. American Nurses' Association: Standards of Nursing Practice. Kansas City, MO, The American Nurses' Association, 1973
21. Bird B: Psychological aspects of preoperative and postoperative care. Am J Nurs 55: 685–687, 1955
22. Joint Commission on Accreditation of Hospitals: Accreditation Manual for Hospitals. Chicago, Joint Commission on Accreditation for Hospitals, 1981
23. Devine EC, Cook TD: A meta-analytic analysis of effects of psychoeducational interventions on length of post-surgical hospital stay. Nurs Res 32: 267–274, 1983
24. Dison C, Kinnaird L: Negotiating a patient teaching policy in the community hospital. Nurs Admin Q 4: 13–17, 1980
25. Minnick A: Patient teaching by registered nurses: A study of the relationship of beliefs, intentions, and health locus of control with teaching behavior. Unpublished doctoral dissertation, Northwestern University, 1981

11

Effective Time Management

ONE OF an individual's most important work resources is one's time. While everyone has the same amount and it cannot be stockpiled in advance or saved, people differ significantly in the way they manage this critical commodity. Those who succeed tend to be more productive, more satisfied, less stressed, and more healthy than others.

Time management can be defined as the application of the basic management skills of planning, organizing, directing, and controlling to the individual's own work activities.[1] Since time is a constant and cannot itself be managed, the primary focus is on managing the manner in which one uses time.

The importance of time management in nursing has long been recognized. It is an area over which nurses exercise a relatively high degree of voluntary control; in other words, the specific way that a nurse uses time is mostly a matter of conscious choice. Although this is not always true, it is generally the case that nurses have discretionary control over their time. Thus, nurses must learn to efficiently manage their use of time. The importance of assertive self-management was emphasized by

McConnell,[2] who convincingly pointed out that if the nurse does not manage her own time, someone else will do it for her.

In an excellent article about neonatal intensive care units, Brown argued that a smoothly functioning nursing unit requires good time management.[3] She asserted that the "tyranny of the urgent," frequent disruptions, and constant changes can only be overcome by effectively managing one's time. McConnell noted that time management actually facilitates the attainment of humanistic goals in nursing and leads directly to significant improvements in the quality of patient care.[2]

Time management continues to be one of the most popular topics in nursing, as well as in business. An article in the Wall Street Journal indicated that time management is the third most popular area of employee training, following orientation and performance appraisal.[4] Fully 74% of all organizations with more than 50 employees regularly offer internal or in-house courses on time management.

Numerous excellent books and articles have been written on the subject. A partial listing of the most frequently cited sources in nursing and health care follows: Applebaum and Rohrs,[5] McConnell,[2] Morano,[6] Norville,[7] Rutkowski,[8] and Schwartz and Mackenzie.[9] Excellent general management sources include the works by Ashkenas and Schaffer,[10] Douglass and Douglass,[11] Lakein,[12] Mackenzie,[13] Schilit,[14] Turla and Hawkins,[15] and Webber.[16]

Although the role of effective time management in nursing has been addressed by many writers, recent changes in the profession have further emphasized the critical nature of this topic. For example, the trends toward complete RN staffing and increased patient loads, combined with the emphasis on cost-effectiveness, make it imperative that nurses at all levels learn to manage their time more efficiently.

In the future, fewer, better educated nurses will be required to do more with less. Given that time is money and complete RN staffs are relatively expensive, nurses must adapt and work smarter in (1) accomplishing their mission and (2) containing staffing expenditures. The ultimate success of these efforts depends on the effective use of time. The message is clear; future improvements in the cost-effectiveness of nursing practice will require efficient time management at all levels.

The purpose of this chapter is to provide an introduction to the topic of time management and a general overview of the available literature. In addition, based on a review of the research and writing in both nursing and management, a comprehensive seven-step model leading to improved time management is presented.

MAJOR OBSTACLES TO EFFECTIVE TIME MANAGEMENT

Several major obstacles or "time robbers" exist which make effective time management a difficult proposition. Although countless potential difficulties exist, in this section the most common, frequently mentioned problems are briefly addressed. As you read through them, reflect on how many of them apply to you personally and how serious they are. People with chronic time management problems tend to illustrate a pattern of misuse involving several of these obstacles.

Lack of Priorities

People who have trouble managing their time effectively often lack a clear understanding of their work priorities. They do not view their job as a set of prioritized tasks differing in terms of their significance and they do not approach the job by addressing the high priority tasks first.

Rather than responding to the job in a productive, well-planned manner, time wasters spend the day responding to crises. The work day involves moving from one emergency to the next, with no underlying plan or set of objectives. By the end of the day, the nurse might have worked very hard and done a lot, but important tasks and responsibilities have typically been overlooked or neglected in the process.

Indecisiveness/Procrastination

The job of being a nurse or nurse manager involves making decisions and taking action. Indecisiveness and procrastination can severely limit a nurse's effectiveness and can cripple her ability to accomplish all required work tasks efficiently. The time spent in delaying a decision or postponing required action is time lost to the nurse, making it even more difficult to meet all major responsibilities.

Inability to Delegate

This problem of delegation of work plagues many nurse managers, especially new supervisors. Rather than appropriately assigning task responsibility and authority to subordinates, managers often keep too much of the work for themselves. Reasons for this are numerous and include (1) a lack of supervisory training in how to delegate properly, (2) insecurity on the part of the manager, (3) a lack of trust, (4) a belief that the manager can do it quicker and better, and (5) a feeling that subordinates will resent the assignments and responsibility.

Managers who fail to delegate attempt to do everything themselves, including unimportant tasks. Since in most situations it is impossible to do everything well, important tasks are often either not completed or done in a hurried, unsatisfactory manner. Unfortunately, in such situations, job stress is a likely consequence.

Perfectionism and Excessive Attention to Detail

This problem is often associated with the inability to delegate work to subordinates. It involves almost an obsession with perfection and attention to minute detail in all tasks, including trivial ones. Although high standards of quality work are certainly desirable in any nurse, overconcern with exacting precision and perfection can reduce time available for more important work and can substantially detract from overall effectiveness.

Inefficient Meetings

In most organizations, work-related meetings constitute one of the most pervasive time wasters. A survey reported in Time indicated that managers spend an average of 16.5 hours/week in meetings, with one third of those sessions considered unnecessary by the people involved.[17] It seems that the principal problem is the typical regularly scheduled meetings at which nothing is accomplished.

Nurses, and especially nurse managers, spend a great deal of their time in meetings of various types. How many of these meetings are actually essential to the accomplishment of basic nursing functions and how much time is wasted even in necessary meetings? Remember that time is money. With six people in a meeting, wasting 30 minutes results in the loss of 3 valuable hours of nursing service and makes it more difficult for those people to get their own work done.

Telephone Interruptions

How many times have you been concentrating and working on an important project, report, or memo, only to be interrupted by a routine telephone call? Typically, after handling such a call, it is not easy to return immediately to your tasks and continue to work efficiently. This is even more problematic when multiple telephone interruptions occur. Frequent routine telephone calls can destroy a person's ability to concentrate and work well and can represent a major obstacle to effective time management.

Drop-in Visitors and Non-Job-Related Conversation

How often do people come to your office or work area to talk about something that may or may not be job related? Offending visitors can include friends from other units or departments, co-workers, subordinates, or even supervisors. These interruptions can substantially interfere with a nurse's work, making it difficult to complete tasks in a timely manner. When the focus of the conversation is on something other than the nurse's major work priorities, the visit constitutes a waste of time. Unfortunately, over the course of a week, many hours are typically lost in such irrelevant visits and conversations.

Smoking/Coffee Ritual

If you smoke or drink coffee or have observed others engaged in these behaviors at work, you are aware of the smoking/coffee ritual. With smokers, the process begins by searching for cigarettes, a light, and an ashtray. It continues with lighting the cigarette, puffing and smoking it, discarding the ash, and finally extinguishing it. The same steps are followed each time the person smokes.

Although one can smoke at one's desk or work station, the coffee ritual typically involves walking to wherever the drink is available. The process includes searching for a cup, the coffee, creamer, sugar, and stirrer. Then one returns to the office or work area and drinks until the cup is empty, at which point the process can begin again. It might also be necessary occasionally to actually brew the coffee, which can be a time-consuming task.

Depending on the frequency of consumption of cigarettes or coffee, considerable time can be wasted during a day. In some extreme cases, as much as 1 to 2 hours can be wasted daily. If this amount of time sounds high, monitor your own behavior or that of others engaged in smoking or coffee drinking and record the time involved. You will probably be surprised by the result.

Inability to Say No

The final major obstacle to effective time management involves a nurse's inability to assertively refuse special non-job-related requests from friends, co-workers, subordinates, supervisors, patients, and family members. There are only so many hours in the day and time spent dealing with special projects leaves less time available for the significant aspects of one's work. Although everyone likes to be perceived as a helpful person, and a certain amount of volunteer assistance improves one's work and interpersonal effectiveness, frequent involvement in non-job-related activities can quickly overwhelm the nurse and can leave less time for essential functions.

COMPREHENSIVE APPROACH TO TIME MANAGEMENT IMPROVEMENT

Based on a review of the various time management techniques, strategies, and advice available in the nursing and management literatures, a comprehensive seven-step approach to time utilization improvement was developed. The model is designed as a systematic framework for enhancing individual time management.

The seven-step process is illustrated in the box, Comprehensive Seven-Step Approach to Successful Time Management.

TIME PERSPECTIVE/ATTITUDE SELF-ASSESSMENT

People have different perspectives and attitudes toward time and how they use or manage it. These differences are a function of such interrelated factors as culture, personality, upbringing, and occupational background. Some people rush through life, doing everything in a frenzied manner, whereas others approach life in

---

**COMPREHENSIVE SEVEN-STEP APPROACH
TO SUCCESSFUL TIME MANAGEMENT**

---

1. Time perspective/attitude self-assessment of one's perspective or attitude toward time and time management
2. Detailed analysis of one's work priorities or objectives
3. Time/activities audit to determine how one is spending the work day
4. Mastery of time management techniques
5. Development and implementation of a personal time management strategy, which includes a combination of techniques that work best for the individual
6. Monitor and measure performance improvement by completing a second time/activities audit and comparing it to the first one
7. Self-motivation to reward successes and reinforce new habits

---

a deliberate, or even lazy manner. The optimal approach, as with most things, lies somewhere in between these two extremes.

Your perspective and attitude toward time are important determinants of your success in managing it effectively. Certain perspectives and attitudes can be assets, whereas others make it difficult to manage time well. Some indication of where you are placed on these dimensions can be helpful in beginning the process of improving your own personal time management.

Two useful self-assessment questionnaires are available that can offer valuable insights into your perspective and attitude toward time and its use. These measures are designed to give a general indication of your orientation and are not rigorously developed psychological instruments.

Complete the two questionnaires and then review the scoring interpretation. The information and insights you gain will hopefully help you to understand yourself better and show you how to approach your management of time.

The first survey, the Time Perspective Self-Analysis, and the assocated interpretational guidelines are adopted from Roseman.[18] This instrument is provided in Figure 11-1. Respond to each of the 20 items by checking "Yes" or "No." Answer the questions quickly and be honest with yourself. Once you are finished, continue with the interpretational guidelines.

The Time Perspective Self-Analysis was designed to identify three basic perspectives or attitudes toward time: urgency, concern, and self-criticism. The Urgency Scale includes items 3, 6, 7, 10, and 12 and two distinct patterns are possible. Pattern U-1 consists of the following item responses:

Item 3 — Yes
Item 6 — Yes
Item 7 — Yes
Item 10 — No
Item 12 — Yes

	Yes	No
1. Are you concerned about wasting time?	____	____
2. Do you wish you had more time?	____	____
3. Do you want to be on time?	____	____
4. Do you make the most of your time?	____	____
5. Can you find time for important things?	____	____
6. Do you want to save time?	____	____
7. Do you feel the pressure of time?	____	____
8. Do you spend your time wisely?	____	____
9. Do you wait until the last minute?	____	____
10. Do you have plenty of time?	____	____
11. Do you put things off until another time?	____	____
12. Do you rush projects because of time pressure?	____	____
13. Is your time well organized?	____	____
14. Do others rob your time?	____	____
15. Do you have free time?	____	____
16. Are you trying to do too much at one time?	____	____
17. Are you realistic in setting time deadlines?	____	____
18. Are you in control of your time?	____	____
19. Do you have the time to think?	____	____
20. Have you tried to change your time habits?	____	____

FIGURE 11-1. *Time perspective self-analysis.*

It suggests that you are in the proper frame of mind to undertake a time management improvement program. You have a powerful sense of time urgency and time pressures are causing major problems in your life. Thus, your motivation to make an improvement is strong.

On the other hand, Pattern U-2 indicates little feeling of urgency about time or time management. This pattern is represented by the following item responses:

Item   3 — No
Item   6 — No
Item   7 — No
Item 10 — Yes
Item 12 — No

Without a compelling sense of time urgency, you are unlikely to be seriously interested in managing your time better. Generally, you lack the motivation necessary to begin an improvement program or make it work.

The second basic attitude measured by the Time Perspective Self-Analysis is represented by the Concern Scale, which includes items 1, 2, 4, 9, 11, 14, 15, and 19. Again, two separate patterns are possible in this scale. Pattern C-1 is evidenced by the following item responses:

Item   1 — Yes
Item   2 — Yes
Item   4 — Yes
Item   9 — No
Item 11 — No
Item 14 — Yes
Item 15 — No
Item 19 — No

It indicates that you have a genuine concern about managing your time effectively and places a high value on improvement efforts. Combined with a sense of time urgency, this attitude is critical to the success of any attempt to improve personal time management.

Conversely, Pattern C-2 represents an attitude that actually interferes with effective time management. It is reflected in the following item responses:

Item 1 — No
Item 2 — No
Item 4 — No
Item 9 — Yes
Item 11 — Yes
Item 14 — No
Item 15 — Yes
Item 19 — Yes

This pattern suggests that you have minimal concern for managing your time well and place little value on improvement in this area. Under these circumstances effective time management is almost impossible.

The third and final component of the Time Perspective Self-Analysis is known as the Self-Criticism Scale. This scale includes items 5, 8, 13, 16, 17, 18, and 20, and also consists of two different patterns. The following item responses make up Pattern S-1:

Item 5 — No
Item 8 — No
Item 13 — No
Item 16 — Yes
Item 17 — No
Item 18 — No
Item 20 — No

This pattern suggests that you are already aware of your major problems relating to your management of time. You recognize where your weaknesses are and you have a high level of accurate self-insight. Consequently, you are likely to benefit greatly from improvement efforts designed to address your deficiencies.

Pattern S-2 consists of the following item responses:

Item 5 — Yes
Item 8 — Yes
Item 13 — Yes
Item 16 — No
Item 17 — Yes

Item 18 — Yes

Item 20 — Yes

Two different interpretations are possible with this pattern. If you were frank, honest, and accurate in completing the scale, an S-2 pattern suggests that you are already managing your time well and that you have no serious problems.

If, on the other hand, you were less than honest with yourself and your responses were not accurate, the S-2 pattern indicates that you are unaware of or not willing to admit that you have major time management problems. A lack of accurate self-awareness obviously makes it difficult to see the need for improvement in this area.

The aforementioned three scales represent basic perspectives or attitudes toward time and time management. If your own responses do not fit perfectly into any of the patterns, you probably fall somewhere in between the basic categories. Thus, you should modify your interpretation of the explanatory guidelines accordingly.

The ideal candidate for a time management improvement program is one with a strong sense of time urgency (Pattern U-1), a genuine concern for effective time management (Pattern C-1), and an accurate level of self-criticism (Pattern S-1). People with other combinations on these three patterns are less likely to be successful in improving their management of time until fundamental attitudinal changes occur.

The second instrument that can be useful in understanding one's orientation toward time is based on the work of Friedman and Rosenman.[19] This questionnaire is given in Figure 11-2. Take a few minutes and respond to each of the eight items using the 1-5 scale from "Rarely" to "Almost Always." Answer rapidly and as honestly as possible. Continue with the interpretation when you are finished.

Friedman and Rosenman conducted basic research on the relationship between personality and heart disease.[19] They found that certain personality types are more prone to heart problems than others. The scale in Figure 11-2 provides a simple measure of two basic personality orientations that relate to the use of time and subsequent heart disease known as Type A and Type B.

In order to get a general indication of what personality type you have, add up your responses to the eight items and divide by

Instructions

The questions below relate to your personality and your perspective on time. Read each question. Pause to think about your typical behavior in each situation and then check (✓) the appropriate response. When you have finished, return to where you stopped reading in the text.

	Rarely 1	Sometimes 2	Often 3	Most of the time 4	Almost always 5
1. Do you speak rapidly and grow impatient when talking with others who speak slowly?	( )	( )	( )	( )	( )
2. Do you quickly grow impatient when in slow traffic, standing in line, or when waiting for someone?	( )	( )	( )	( )	( )
3. Do you eat, walk, and do other day-to-day tasks rapidly?	( )	( )	( )	( )	( )
4. Do you complete more than one task simultaneously (e.g., working while watching TV; writing a note while someone is talking to you)?	( )	( )	( )	( )	( )
5. Do you compete against fellow workers or against yourself to meet a quota of work or a time deadline?	( )	( )	( )	( )	( )
6. Do you feel uneasy or vaguely guilty when you are not working for extended periods?	( )	( )	( )	( )	( )
7. Do you deny yourself enjoyment in order to complete goals and rationalize this behavior by promising that you will relax when the goals have been achieved?	( )	( )	( )	( )	( )
8. Do you tightly schedule life's activities including work, regular leisure time, and vacations?	( )	( )	( )	( )	( )

FIGURE 11-2. *Personality and the concept of time.*

eight. If most of your answers are 4 ("most of the time") or 5 ("almost always"), and your average score is above three, you tend to exhibit a Type A personality.

This is characterized by an aggressive, incessant struggle to accomplish more in less time. The Type A person constantly rushes to accomplish tasks, often engages in two or more activities simultaneously, and is a victim of "hurry sickness" as described by Friedman and Rosenman.[19] Extreme Type A behavior has been linked with heart disease and a host of other stress-related problems.

If most of your responses are 1 ("rarely") or 2 ("sometimes"), and your average score is less than three, you tend to exhibit a Type B personality and are not driven by an obsession with time and constant activity. Research has shown that Type B persons are significantly less likely to develop cardiac problems than Type A individuals.

Most people are not extreme Type As or Bs, but fall somewhere in between. As indicated in the interpretation of the Time Perspective Self-Analysis, a certain degree of urgency and concern about time and its use are necessary before a successful improvement program can be initiated. However, as the research by Friedman and Rosenman has demonstrated, an obsession with time can have a negative impact on one's health.[19] Thus, the "optimal" personality orientation towards time involves a blend of both Type A and Type B behaviors.

ANALYSIS OF WORK PRIORITIES

After learning something about yourself and your time perspective and attitude, the second step in the model involves a systematic work priorities analysis. An individual must clearly understand what her major work tasks and responsibilities are, along with their relative importance. This information should be formulated ideally in conjunction with one's supervisor, resulting in a listing of the major dimensions of one's job together with associated percentage weights indicating relative importance. The topic of clarifying performance expectations is a central issue in performance appraisal and is more fully discussed in Chapter 6.

An old adage states that "If you don't know where you are going, any road will take you there." Nothing is more true about effective time management. Unless you know what you should be doing on your job, or where you want to be directing your efforts, work activities of any kind will make you feel as if something is being accomplished.

In business management, the Pareto Principle states that 80% of the impact you have in your job is achieved by 20% of the actual work activities. Thus, one must identify the high priority tasks in one's job so that they can be addressed first. Again, with no priorities, one activity is perceived as just as valuable and useful as another. Unfortunately, this does not accurately reflect the reality present in most jobs.

Consequently, a clear written summary of one's major performance dimensions and their relative importance is essential in developing a comprehensive program to improve time management. The written work priorities should serve ideally as a set

Instructions
Read the questions in Parts I and II carefully. Think about your present
habits and practices relating to how you use your time, and place a check (✓)
in the appropriate column. When you have completed both Parts I and II,
add all the numbered values assigned to the questions in Part I and divide
by eight then do likewise for Part II. When you have finished, return to
where you stopped reading in the text.

Part I

	Rarely 1	Sometimes 2	Often 3	Most of the time 4	Almost always 5
1. Do you tend to tackle the short, simple, pleasant tasks of your job before the difficult more time-consuming tasks?	( )	( )	( )	( )	( )
2. How often do you fail to plan because you don't feel you can take the time?	( )	( )	( )	( )	( )
3. How often do you set objectives for a particular day and then find that at the end of the day you have not accomplished them?	( )	( )	( )	( )	( )
4. How often do you find yourself responding to what others consider urgent rather than doing what you feel is important?	( )	( )	( )	( )	( )
5. How often do you become angry at yourself for having agreed to do something that you really didn't want to do?	( )	( )	( )	( )	( )
6. How often do you find yourself engaging in details and activities rather than focusing on results and contributions to the organization?	( )	( )	( )	( )	( )
7. How often do you find yourself sacrificing leisure or family time in order to do your job?	( )	( )	( )	( )	( )
8. How often do you miss important deadlines in your work?	( )	( )	( )	( )	( )

(continued)

FIGURE 11-3. *Time management practices.*

of objectives to guide work efforts and provide a means of evaluating whether one's time is being used optimally.

TIME/ACTIVITIES AUDIT

Once a systematic work priorities analysis has been completed, the next step in the program to improve time management is the completion of a time/activities audit. This is designed to identify how you are currently spending your time and where any problems exist.

A preliminary indication of how well you are presently managing your time can be obtained by completing the questionnaire contained in Figure 11-3. This measure was originally developed by Norville.[6]

				Most of	Almost
Part II					
	Rarely	Sometimes	Often	the time	always
	1	2	3	4	5
1. Do you schedule your most difficult tasks at a time when your level of personal energy tends to be high?	( )	( )	( )	( )	( )
2. How often do you take time to analyze the content of your job to determine whether you can combine, delegate, or eliminate certain activities?	( )	( )	( )	( )	( )
3. How often do you set aside segments of time and control interruptions in order to focus on important work?	( )	( )	( )	( )	( )
4. Do you keep a brief written record of how you use your time at work and review it periodically for insights?	( )	( )	( )	( )	( )
5. How often do you establish written priorities, budget your time in advance to complete them, and maintain a daily "to do" list?	( )	( )	( )	( )	( )
6. How often do you take time to segment similar activities in completing your daily work?	( )	( )	( )	( )	( )
7. How often do you set measurably verifiable objectives in advance of meetings that are your responsibility rather than simply preparing an agenda?	( )	( )	( )	( )	( )
8. How often do you analyze your work environment to identify people or processes that contribute to ineffectiveness in using the time available?	( )	( )	( )	( )	( )

FIGURE 11-3. *(continued)*

Complete Sections I and II, using the 1–5 scale from "rarely" to "almost always." Place a check in the appropriate column, work quickly, and respond as honestly and as accurately as possible. Return to the following interpretational information when you finish.

You should first compute your overall scores for Sections I and II separately. Do this by adding up the eight individual item scores in each section. Total scores can range from a low of 8 to a high of 40.

Section I addresses ineffective time management practices. A high score, between 30 and 40, indicates poor time management, while a low score of 8 to 18 suggests that you are able to successfully avoid many of the most common pitfalls. Scores in the mid-range from 19 to 29 reflect moderate problems in managing time well.

The eight items in Section II deal with effective practices. In this case, a high score (30 to 40) is very positive and associated with sound time management. A low score, from 8 to 18, indicates a lack of familiarity with or use of effective techniques, whereas a mid-range score, from 19 to 29, is associated with a moderate level of success in managing one's time. Clearly, the ideal pattern is a combination of a very low score in Section I and a very high score in Section II. Your score on these two sections will provide a general indication of how well you are currently managing your time.

However, if you are serious about improvement in this area, you must complete a time/activities audit. This requirement is universally recommended by writers and researchers in time management. It involves keeping a record or log of your daily work activities for 2 to 3 weeks.

Although this activity can itself be time consuming and burdensome, it is critical to the success of any time management improvement strategy. Typically, individuals are unaware of exactly how they spend their time at work, what their major activities really are, and where problems exist. The time/activities log provides invaluable data in analyzing time use patterns and identifying major problem areas. An interesting example of the development, implementation, and use of a time/activities log in nursing is provided in an article by Lucas and Austin.[20]

To facilitate the process of recording your daily activities, a sample Time/Activities Log is provided in Figure 11-4. It should be completed on a daily basis for 2 to 3 weeks. The form consists of two kinds of activities: (1) routine ones performed on a regular basis and (2) nonroutine tasks performed irregularly. Beginning at the start of a shift, you should record your activities over the course of the day, indicating the times that you start and stop and checking the appropriate activity engaged in.

Invariably, maintaining this record will change the way you spend your time. Nevertheless, try to behave as you normally would at work.

After recording a daily log for 2 to 3 weeks, you should have enough data to begin the process of examining how you spend your time and what your problems are. The analysis of this information consists of three separate components: overall time usage, work priorities' comparison, and problem identification.

Name: _____

Date: _____

Time period		Activities									Other: specify									
		Routine																		
Start	Stop	Vital signs	Dispense medicine	Patient teaching	Recording or charting	Meeting	Telephone	Patient or family	Meal time	Break										

FIGURE 11-4. *Sample time/activities log.*

Overall Time Usage

This component involves totaling up all time spent on both job-related and non-job-related activities and computing the percentage of time spent on each. For example, over a 2-week period of 40 hours/week, a total of 80 hours are worked. If 60 hours are spent on job-related tasks, a total of 60/80 or 75% of one's time is spent constructively, while 20/80 or 25% is wasted or mismanaged. These percentages will give you an overall and fairly accurate indication of how well you are managing your time. In most cases, people are shocked to discover the extent to which they waste time each week.

Comparison of Work Priorities

In this analysis, a person's work priorities (as developed in Step 2) are compared to the actual use of work time. Time should ideally be managed so as to correspond closely to work priorities. For instance, if a nurse has patient teaching as one of her major performance dimensions, with a relative importance weight of 40%, time spent on this activity should equal approximately 40% of the available work hours. If the time/activities log indicates that only 20% of total hours is being spent in patient teaching, a significant problem exists, and efforts to increase teaching hours, while reducing hours spent on other activities, should be initiated.

In a similar manner, the nurse should compare work priorities and their respective percentage weights with actual time spent on those activities. Corrective strategies are required where major differences exist. For most nurses, this type of analysis will reveal substantial discrepancies between what they should be doing or what they think they are doing and what is actually being done.

Problem Identification

This analysis entails a detailed evaluation of the non-work-related entries recorded in the time/activities log. Each such activity should be listed along with the total and percentage time spent. A review of this list will indicate what the individual's major time-wasting activities are. Further analysis of these activities should reveal which ones are under the direct control or discretion of the nurse and which are not. Attention should then be directed to addressing the major problem areas over which the nurse exercises control.

The time/activities log, if completed and analyzed thoroughly, can provide the nurse with crucial information in identifying and defining patterns of time management and salient problem areas. As such, completion of the log is an essential step in any systematic program to improve the management of one's time.

The initial time/activities log should be saved for use as a baseline comparison with a similar log that should be completed after implementing a time management strategy. This is the only means of objectively determining if improvements have actually been made.

TIME MANAGEMENT STRATEGIES

After completing the time/activities log and analyzing the data, the next step involves learning about the various time management techniques that are available. Based on a review of the nursing and management literatures, several approaches to time management can be identified. In this section, these approaches are individually presented and briefly discussed. Although many of the specific techniques are commonly mentioned by multiple authors, when applicable, unique approaches are credited to the original source.

Assertiveness and Politeness

In managing one's time effectively, it is important and often essential to be assertive with others, including co-workers, subordinates, supervisors, friends, and family. Since work success depends on the sound management of time, you have every right to assertively pursue more efficient time use strategies. However, it is also important to be polite and considerate, so as not to unnecessarily alienate anyone.

List Making

Based on the work priorities' analysis completed in step two of the time management improvement model, an individual should be able to list major work goals or objectives for the following year. This written list should be displayed prominently in the work area to serve as a ready reminder of what needs to be accomplished.

Once annual goals have been established, it is then possible to work backwards and formulate specific monthly and weekly sub-goals that must be attained in order to achieve the annual ones. This process should continue by developing a daily list of specific objectives, keeping in mind the weekly, monthly, and yearly goals.

Although some writers suggest that the daily list of projects to be done should be completed during the first 10 to 15 minutes of the work day, it is generally recommended that this list be generated the day before, prior to leaving work. In this manner, the plan for the following day is established, thus allowing for an immediate mobilization of effort when the next work day begins.

Most people find that crossing items off on this list is a satisfying and motivating experience and gives them a sense of accomplishment. The potency of this seemingly simple act was emphasized at a seminar by a manager who reported that when she completed something important that had been inadvertently left off her list of things to do, she added it anyway in order to be able to cross it off.

Everyone, at all levels in an organization, should be encouraged to use such a list. The list facilitates the process of organizing, prioritizing, and accomplishing one's work. The likelihood that important tasks will be neglected is also minimized.

Knowledge of Yourself

It is important that people know themselves and when they work best. Difficult or thoughtful work should be scheduled for peak periods, with less demanding activities during other times. For example, a "morning person" should ideally tackle the tough tasks during the early hours of the day, reserving easier, routine work for later. The opposite is true for an "afternoon person." By knowing yourself and when you work best, individuals can significantly improve their personal productivity and efficient use of time.

Uninterrupted Quiet Time

If possible, the nurse or nurse manager should reserve uninterrupted blocks of quiet time during the day to deal with creative, thoughtful, or difficult tasks. The absence of disturbances allows for greater concentration and efficiency in completing work activities. Charting, for example, is often best done in a quiet place and not at the nurses' station. Preparing budgets or performance appraisals are managerial tasks that require concentration and thought, and are thus also best accomplished during quiet, uninterrupted periods of time.

A unit or personal secretary can be invaluable in screening visitors and calls to allow for undisturbed work time. Everyone should try to reserve at least 1 or 2 hours each day to devote to their most important tasks.

Orderly Work Area

An orderly, well-maintained office or work area can be a useful tool in reducing time spent looking for misplaced important paperwork or items. If you have ever frantically searched through a messy office for a critical memorandum or piece of equipment, you can appreciate the value of this suggestion.

Personal Filing System

The organization and retrieval of important work-related information is greatly facilitated by a simple personal filing system consisting of folders for major topical areas. Common examples include out-going correspondence, incoming hospital/departmental/unit communication, upcoming events, and new nursing techniques or procedures.

The files should be labeled clearly and maintained in alphabetical order. Any correspondence or printed information pertaining to a particular topic should be filed in the appropriate folder. Thus, when needed, all relevant data are readily available in one place.

A personal filing system helps one organize work-related information systematically and reduces the time needed to locate it.

In addition, a 30-day suspense file can help keep track of significant upcoming events and obligations. It consists of three sets of file folders: (a) 31 folders representing the days in a month, (b) 12 folders for each of the months in the year, and (c) two folders for the succeeding 2 years. Noteworthy activities and commitments are recorded on paper and filed in the appropriate folder. When a new month begins, the material in the monthly folder is then distributed to the daily folders. In this manner, one has a convenient record of important events for each day of the present month, as well as future months in the year and the next 2 years. A personal 30-day suspense file can be an invaluable aid in organizing and managing one's time effectively.

Processing of Paperwork

A helpful time management technique involves the use of a six-category approach to processing paperwork that includes the following: (a) requires immediate attention, (b) save for later action, (c) give to someone else for review or action, (d) save for later reading, (e) place in personal files, and (f) throw away. Ideally, incoming paperwork should be reviewed quickly and placed in the appropriate category. This ensures that all material is initially seen and important tasks can be identified for immediate action. Once the classification process is completed, one can quickly begin work on the high priority tasks requiring a timely response.

Concentration on One Task at a Time

For most people, maximum work efficiency is attained by concentrating one's effort on a single task, rather than attempting to deal with many tasks simultaneously. One should sharply focus effort and attention on the task at hand until completed and then begin another.

This is especially true with routine tasks, which often tend to be left unfinished. Thus, for example, it is advisable to complete the charting, dispose of all used needles, and clean up messes when they occur, rather than saving these tasks for later. Try to avoid creating a back log of unfinished jobs that can lead to confusion, oversight, error, and inefficiency.

Grouping of Similar Tasks

This technique does not involve working on tasks simultaneously, but rather grouping tasks together in terms of their similarity and then dealing with them one at a time. For example, if a nurse manager has a series of budget-related tasks to do, it is recommended that they be done together instead of separately. Using this approach, information relevant to budgetary matters is only assembled once for use in dealing with all of the related tasks, thus resulting in the efficient use and conservation of time.

Intermediate Goals For Long Projects

Everyone is faced occasionally with major work projects that might take weeks or months to complete. In such situations, it is advisable to break the project down into shorter term, intermediate subtasks that can be more easily addressed. Initial success in accomplishing the subtasks can serve to effectively motivate efforts to finish the overall project.

Starting Difficult Tasks

For most people, it is much easier to neglect or avoid a task that is not started as opposed to one that is incomplete. Consequently, with difficult or undesirable jobs, it is important to start them, even if it is only a small step. By beginning the work effort, you will substantially increase the likelihood that the task will be completed eventually.

Standardization of Routine Reports and Correspondence

Much of the paperwork that nurses and nurse managers must generate is of a routine, recurrent nature. When possible, standardized formats, sentences, or paragraphs should be developed, saved, and used when called for. This reduces the time necessary to reformulate the correspondence each time it is required. Access to a word processor with a memory capacity can greatly facilitate this process.

Selective Reading

Nurses must read a great deal in order to keep up with required departmental/hospital reading and new research and developments in the field. Learning to read selectively and skim effectively can allow a nurse to review important material, extract the key points, and save time in the process. Efforts should be directed at quickly skimming the abstract, summary, or conclusion section of a document to determine if important information is contained in it; if so, more careful consideration and reading is warranted. Written communication formats that help in this regard include the systematic use of one page "executive summaries" for all long reports and limiting internal memos to no more than one page.

Management of Telephone Calls

If possible, routine telephone calls should be screened by a unit or personal secretary. In order to allow for uninterrupted blocks of work time, only important or emergency calls should be immediately dealt with. It is generally recommended that accumulated calls be returned on two occasions, before lunch and before the end of the day.

Restriction of Personal Visits

Drop-in visits by friends, colleagues, or subordinates should be assertively, yet considerately discouraged. You should clearly communicate that you have important work that must be done and that routine matters can be dealt with later on. This is especially important with subordinates who should be instructed not to spontaneously bring routine problems and questions to the supervisor. Important issues and emergencies must, however, be dealt with immediately.

Decisiveness

Nurses and nurse managers must know how to effectively make decisions in order to be successful. As pointed out earlier, indecisiveness and procrastination are major time management obstacles confronting many nurses. When faced with an important decision, nurses should use the following steps in the recommended problem solving or decision making process: (a) collect information necessary to understand and analyze the situation or problem, (b) generate a list of potential strategies or solutions, (c) rationally evaluate each of the options, (d) select the "best" one, (e) implement the decision or solution, and (f) evaluate the impact of the action and make any required modifications.

Timely decisions are a necessity in nursing. Follow the aforementioned process described and do not be afraid to make a decision. With especially critical matters, give yourself a time limit to thoroughly go through the necessary steps and arrive at a sound solution. This might include "sleeping-on" the decision for a few days. When the time limit is up, make the decision, implement it, and do not second guess yourself.

Effective Operation of Meetings

One of the major wastes of time is attending poorly run or unnecessary meetings. In order to deal with this problem, nurses should attempt to operate meetings as effectively as possible. General guidelines include (a) providing the purpose, agenda, and time limit in written form to all participants prior to the meeting, (b) requiring and expecting group member preparation, (c) starting the meeting at the designated time, (d) selecting a meeting coordinator to monitor the group process and adherence to the agenda and time limit, (e) restricting extraneous discussion and comments, and (f) complying with the time limit by stopping on time. Following these suggestions will increase the probability that meetings are efficient, productive, and successful.

Commitments to Others and Cooperation

One powerful way to motivate yourself to accomplish a particularly difficult or undesirable task is to involve others in the process and make mutual commitments concerning what each person will do. By committing yourself and involving other people, it is more difficult to avoid completing a job. The expectations of others can thus serve as a strong incentive to accomplish what has been promised.

Development and Familiarity with Standard Procedures

The development and use of standard operating procedures or protocols to handle routine matters, problems, or DRGs can be an excellent way to improve time management, efficiency, and productivity. Initially, this strategy requires a substantial investment of time and effort to develop optimal methods of addressing common work situations, but the rewards are significant. The use of such standard methods promotes consistency and work quality and allows nurses to complete common tasks in a more timely manner.

Brown has recommended that frequently used standard nursing procedures, telephone numbers, basic assessment outlines, admission orders, laboratory values, and drug information be recorded on index cards or in a pocket notebook and carried at all times.[3] This would prevent the problem of having to look for the needed information and facilitate more rapid response times. In addition, Brown advised that supplies and equipment be kept in standardized locations, familiar to everyone. Thus, time spent searching for these materials would be minimized.

Delegation of Work to Subordinates

This technique is appropriate for nurse managers who exercise supervisory authority over others. One of the most useful managerial skills involves delegating work responsibility and authority to competent, well trained, trustworthy subordinates, thus allowing the supervisor to devote more time and energy to primary responsibilities. Effective delegation requires the following components: (a) a concerted effort on the part of the supervisor to properly train and develop subordinates, providing them with the skills necessary to make decisions effectively and take action, (b) assigning decision-making authority to subordinates that is commensurate with the responsibility involved, (c) promoting a strong degree of trust between supervisor and subordinate, and (d) establishing a feedback system to monitor decisions made by subordinates.

Delegating work to subordinates helps them to grow and develop their managerial and decision-making skills. It also tends to enhance job challenge and promote work satisfaction. From the manager's perspective, delegation allows for the accomplishment of more work in an efficient manner and conserves valuable time and energy for high priority tasks.

Unit or Group Meetings

Periodically, it can be useful to conduct unit or group meetings for the purpose of discussing and sharing various time management techniques. This encourages involvement and commitment and can often result in several excellent suggestions for improvement.

Effective Use of Slack, Idle, or Waiting Time

How often have you had to wait for an extended time in one of the following situations: (a) holding for someone on the telephone, (b) awaiting the start of a meeting, (c) sitting in a doctor or dentist's office, or (d) caught in a traffic jam? Such occurrences are major potential time wasters. However, with proper planning, instances of slack, idle, or waiting time can be effectively put to use. The recommended strategy is to reserve routine, relatively simple tasks for these periods, such as journal or report reading and short memos or letters. The ideal task is one that requires little thought and can be easily started and stopped.

Work of this type should then be taken with you throughout the day. When you are forced into a waiting situation, you can then use the time constructively and avoid the feelings of frustration and stress often associated with imposed idleness. You will also have more time available at work for difficult or thoughtful tasks.

DEVELOPMENT AND IMPLEMENTATION OF A PERSONAL STRATEGY

It should be clear from a review of the specific time management techniques discussed that not all of them will work for everyone. As a unique individual, you will find that some of them will work well and others will not work at all. In this step of the model, the focus is on identifying those techniques that will work best for you and combining them into a comprehensive strategy to improve your time management skills.

From the approaches presented, you should be able to find at least three to four that you could adopt for personal use. As a guide in selecting these procedures, be sure to keep in mind your major time management problems outlined in the time/activities audit. Techniques to address salient problems should ideally be included in your overall strategy.

Once you have developed a well conceived improvement plan, consisting of a set of specific techniques, it should be implemented at work. You should begin to systematically use the new procedures when appropriate on the job. Implementation involves taking your improvement ideas from the conceptual or planning stage and putting them into action.

MONITORING AND MEASURING PERFORMANCE IMPROVEMENT

In order to determine if the personal time management improvement strategy implemented in the preceding step has actually worked, it is necessary to monitor and measure one's performance. The only complete and accurate way to make this determination is to perform a second time/activities' audit. An analysis of this log will provide useful data that can be compared with the results obtained from the initial one.

For example, three basic comparisons between the two logs should be made:

1. Total or percentage time wasted
2. Total or percentage time spent on major work priorities

3. Total or percentage time spent on major non-job-related areas

If your time management improvement program has been successful, you would expect to find that time wasted has declined, time spent on work priorities has increased to desired levels, and time spent in major non-job-related areas has decreased. Significantly different results would indicate that your strategy is not functioning as you intended, and modifications are called for.

This step in the model is important. Without it, one never knows whether the time management improvement techniques really work or not. The answer to this issue is best obtained by completing the second time/activities log and comparing it to the first one. Although this process is time consuming itself, the information you collect is vital to the ultimate success of your improvement program.

SELF-MOTIVATION

The final step in the model to improve time management involves the topic of self-motivation. Unfortunately, this step is missing in most considerations of the subject, yet it is critical to the success of any program. Chapter 5 provides a more in-depth consideration of motivation and incentives, thus only the salient issues as related to time management are discussed here.

Researchers have shown conclusively that people respond to incentives and modify their behavior accordingly. The most direct and powerful incentives are those that are self-administered and independent of other people. This is illustrated in Figure 11-5.

In the first instance, good performance is rewarded by someone other than the individual himself. The relationship between performance and reward is thus dependent on the other person and may or may not be given. In most organizational settings, rewards for good performance are not given as often as they should be. Consequently, the line between good performance and the external reward is dotted, depicting the tenuous nature of the causal relationship.

On the other hand, when good performance is followed by self-reward, the relationship is direct and immediate. The individual knows when he has done a good job and can ensure that

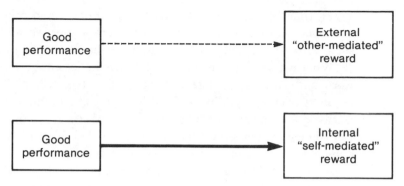

FIGURE 11-5. *External and internal motivation.*

the appropriate reward is forthcoming. Thus, the line between the two is solid, representing the strong causal relationship.

The application of these concepts to time management is straightforward. As an individual, you know when you have done a good job and managed your time well. For most people, although it is easy to fool the boss or others, it is difficult to fool yourself. Therefore, if you are serious about time management, you should regularly reward yourself for successes. Do not wait for someone else to reward you, because this might never happen. When you do well, take the time to recognize your own efforts. As you accomplish your daily objectives, reward yourself for goal attainment.

Many successful people follow this advice on a regular basis. They know what they like and provide self-mediated incentives for good performance. They do not delay gratification, but rather reward themselves during the day and after work. For example, the following have been used by prominent individuals to reward their own good performance during the work day: refreshment breaks, short walks, telephone calls, conversation with friends, light reading, or leisurely lunches. After work, the kinds of self-administered incentives are infinite and include such things as going out to dinner, going out to a movie, watching a favorite television show, relaxing in a hot tub, stopping for a drink, and enjoying time with one's family.

The point is, everyone knows what they like and when they have done a good job that merits a reward. Self-motivation is critical in making a time management program work effectively.

When time is managed well, objectives attained, and problems overcome, self-administered incentives are warranted and will serve to reinforce and motivate similar behavior in the future.

What happens in the case when a person does not do well at work and fails to manage her time well? Is self-punishment required? Generally, the withholding of self-administered rewards is a sufficient deterrent to deal with poor performance. Punishment is not necessary or recommended. If you have not done a good job, simply do not reward yourself.

Although this is straightforward and easy to talk about conceptually, it is difficult and for some people almost impossible to put into practice. Many individuals reward themselves indiscriminately and independent of their performance. In contrast to this approach, the way to successful time management is providing self-administered rewards following good performance and withholding those rewards when you have not done well.

There is an old saying that "you can be your own best friend or your own worst enemy." This is certainly true in relation to time management and self-motivation. If you manage yourself properly, you can dramatically improve your use of time. Poor self-management on the other hand, often characterized by indiscriminate self-reward, will make it difficult to manage your time effectively.

CAVEATS

Before concluding this chapter, several significant caveats must be addressed. Although effective time management is critical to success as a nurse or nurse manager, there are many potential pitfalls associated with improvement efforts.

First, as discussed earlier in the chapter, there are two basic personality orientations with respect to the concept of time. It is certainly possible to become obsessed with efficient time management and adopt many of the Type A behaviors that characterize "hurry sickness."[19] A word of caution is thus in order. Although concern with time is indeed important for success, constantly trying to do too much in too little time is dysfunctional and can lead to a host of serious stress-related problems. Organize and prioritize your efforts and "work smart," but do not push yourself too hard!

Second, in becoming more aware of time and how to manage it, you must realize that you cannot control everything. Unexpected events, emergencies, and special requests or projects can and do occur. Anticipate such occurrences and be flexible in modifying your daily work plan accordingly. Try also to avoid the inevitable feelings of frustration. Your responsibility is to manage the work time that you exercise direct control over. When overriding factors beyond your control dictate how your time is spent, you are not responsible or accountable for the choice of activities. However, when personal control is restored, at that point your time management duties and responsibility begin again.

Finally, be careful to ensure that efforts to improve your time management do not alienate those around you at work. Explain your plan to your co-workers, subordinates, and supervisor, and enlist their cooperation and support. Once you have done this, you should assertively manage your time and guard against major wastes of time. But first, remember to give your colleagues at work the consideration of informing them of your rationale and intentions.

SUMMARY AND CONCLUSIONS

1. Time is one of a nurse's most important resources and thus deserves careful attention and sound management. Current trends toward all RN staffing, increased patient loads, and cost containment make it imperative that nurses at all levels learn to manage their time more effectively.

2. Several major obstacles exist that make it difficult to manage time effectively. Among the most important ones are (a) lack of priorities, (b) indecisiveness/procrastination, (c) inability to delegate, (d) perfectionism and excessive attention to detail, (e) inefficient meetings, (f) telephone interruptions, (g) drop-in visitors and non-job-related conversation, (h) smoking/coffee ritual, and (i) inability to say no.

3. A comprehensive seven-step approach to more effective time management was presented which involves the following components: (a) time perspective/attitude self-assessment, (b) work priorities' analysis, (c) time/activities audit, (d) mastery of time management techniques, (e) development and implementation of a personal time management strategy, (f) monitor and measure success, and (g) self-motivation.

4. One's perspective or attitude toward time is an important determinant of success in managing time effectively. Several useful self-assessment instruments are available. Research with these measures indicates that it is possible to become obsessed with time to the determinant of one's performance and health.

5. In order to manage time successfully, it is necessary to first understand exactly what the requirements and priorities of the job are. Together with one's supervisor, an individual should establish the major dimensions or responsibilities of the job, along with a percentage weight for each one, indicating relative importance.

6. The manner in which a person is currently managing their time is an important consideration in determining how they structure an improvement program. The most comprehensive method available to address this issue is a time/activities audit, which involves recording time spent on all daily activities for 2 to 3 weeks. An analysis of the information will indicate the percentage of time spent on (a) job-related *vs* non-job-related activities, (b) major work priorities, and (c) prominent non-job-related activities.

7. A large number of specific time management techniques have been developed for use. It is helpful to learn about them and try the various approaches in an effort to identify those that work best for the individual.

8. An individualized strategy for time management improvement consists of a combination of specific, personally effective techniques designed to address one's major time-wasting activities and increase productivity and efficiency.

9. In order to evaluate the success of a personal time management improvement strategy, it is necessary to conduct a second time/activities audit and compare it with the initial one. This is the recommended method of determining whether time use patterns have actually improved or not.

10. Time management improvement efforts work best when combined with a systematic program of self-motivation. Individuals should reward themselves for personal successes and withhold rewards following poor performance or mismanagement of time. In this manner, one can motivate and reinforce new, more efficient time use habits.

11. In approaching the issue of time management, one should be aware of three important potential pitfalls: (a) the tendency to become obsessed with time and victimized by "hurry sickness," (b) the failure to recognize that many time-re-

lated and consuming factors are not under an individual's direct control and are thus unmanageable, and (c) the possibility of alienating others at work with overzealous, inconsiderate efforts to strictly manage one's time.

Questions for Reflection and Discussion

1. Why is time considered to be such a critical resource at work? Why is sound time management so important in nursing, especially with the emphasis on cost-effectiveness?

2. What are the major obstacles to effective time management confronting nurses today?

3. What are the strengths and weaknesses of the seven-step approach to time management improvement presented in the chapter and what recommended changes would you suggest?

4. How do nurses typically view time and time management? How does one's perspective or attitude toward time influence the success of improvement efforts?

5. How many nurses clearly understand what their major job priorities are and use them specifically to guide their work behavior? What problems might prevent this from happening?

6. What is a time/activities audit and how should it be analyzed and used in a time management improvement program? In your opinion, what percentage of the average nurse's (nurse manager's) work time is spent on non-job-related activities?

7. Of the various time management techniques presented in the chapter, which are new to you and which do you believe would be new to most nurses? From your experience, can you add any techniques to the list?

8. If you were asked to formulate a personalized time management improvement strategy, what combination of the specific techniques available would you use?

9. What is the best way to determine if a time management improvement strategy has been effective?

10. How do you reward yourself for doing a good job? How often do you regularly reward yourself for effective time management and goal attainment, and how often do you withhold those rewards when you have performed poorly?

11. What are the major potential drawbacks associated with a

time management improvement program? How serious are they in your opinion, and what can be done to deal with them?

REFERENCES

1. Eliopoulous C: Time management: A reminder. J Nurs Admin March, 1984, pp 30–35
2. McConnell E: Ten tactics to help beat the clock. RN Sept 1983, pp 47–50
3. Brown S: Time management: The foundation of a smoothly operating NICU. Neonatal Network October, 1985, pp 44–48
4. Time-management training: For people who can't let their impulses run wild. Wall Street J 16 Aug 1985
5. Applebaum SH, Rohrs WF: Time Management for Health Care Professionals. Rockville, MD, Aspen Systems Corp., 1981
6. Morano VJ: Time management: From victim to victor. The Health Care Supervisor 27: 1–12, 1984
7. Norville JL: Improving personal effectiveness through better management of time. Nursing Homes 13: 8–12, 1984
8. Rutkowski B: Better time management, Nurs Life 4: 53–57, 1984
9. Schwartz EB, Mackenzie RA: Time management strategy for women. J Nurs Admin 9: 22–26, 1979
10. Ashkenas RN, Schaffer RH: Managers can avoid wasting time. Harvard Business Review 60: 99–105, 1982
11. Douglass ME, Douglass DN: Manage Your Time, Manage Your Work, Manage Yourself. New York, AMACOM, 1980
12. Lakein A: How to Get Control of Your Time and Your Life. New York, New American Library, 1973
13. Mackenzie RA: The time trap. New York, AMACOM, 1972
14. Schilit WK: A manager's guide to efficient time management. Personnel J September, 1983, pp 740–747
15. Turla DA, Hawkins KL: Time Management Made Easy. New York, EP Dutton, 1984
16. Webber RA: Time is Money: The Key to Managerial Success. New York, Free Press, 1980
17. This meeting will come to order. Time 16 Dec 1985
18. Roseman E: How to gain control of your time. Prod Man 16: 25–33, 1975
19. Friedman M, Rosenman R: Type A Behavior and Your Heart. New York, Alfred A Knopf, 1974
20. Lucas P, Austin B: The nursing officer at work: Tried and tested. Nurs Times 80: 47–48, 1984

12

Improving Nursing Productivity Through a Regular Physical Fitness Program

INTEREST LEVELS in fitness, health, and wellness in the United States have never been higher. A Gallup Survey, reported in *American Health*,[1] indicates that 69% of all adults are exercising regularly each week (up from 54% 2 years ago). Businesses in the United States have also shown increasing interest in fitness programs for their employees as a way to improve productivity and reduce costs. Higdon reported that over 750 corporations have on-site or in-house fitness facilities, while substantially more companies support programs for employees at local health clubs, gyms, or YWCAs/YMCAs.[2]

In this chapter, the importance of fitness in the nursing profession is examined, along with evidence concerning the potential personal and work-related benefits associated with physical fitness. The role of motivation in facilitating a commitment to fitness is then discussed, followed by an action plan for nursing leaders, designed to promote higher participation rates.

IMPORTANCE AND CURRENT STATUS OF FITNESS IN NURSING

Several writers have emphasized the importance of physical fitness in effectively performing nursing functions.[3-5] Race asserted that few occupations are more physically demanding than nursing and thus high levels of fitness are needed to perform well. Millen has pointed out that a nurse who is physically unfit, not only makes her job more difficult, but also fails to care for patients effectively and often places additional work burdens on other nurses.[4] Clearly, the role of physical fitness in providing quality care is critical.

Physical fitness in nursing is important from another perspective. Brown,[6] Macnamara,[3] and Rimer and Glassman have all identified the special responsibility that nurses have as role models and leaders of the fitness movement.[7] They cogently argue that nurses must demonstrate, by personal example and attitude, their belief in the positive value of fitness. From their perspective, enthusiastic, physically fit nurses are ideally qualified to lead efforts to improve health and fitness levels among both patients and the general public.

Given the obvious importance of fitness in nursing, one might expect to find that most nurses exercise on a regular basis and maintain high levels of personal fitness. Unfortunately, little empirical evidence is available to estimate this figure. Rimer and Glassman conducted a 10-year review of the nursing literature in search of empirical research documenting participation rates and fitness levels.[7] Of the 13 articles they identified, none contained any actual data. Instead, the articles consisted primarily of personal advice on how to start an exercise program or why exercise is important. Nevertheless, Rimer and Glassman speculated that nurses may have been slower to get involved in fitness than other groups in the population. The title of their article was *The Fitness Revolution: Will Nurses Sit This One Out?*

One research study was identified that dealt with fitness levels among female hospital employees, of which most were nurses. Yiasemides assessed the aerobic fitness levels of 64 females in a 120-bed community hospital, using a physical recovery index recommended by the American Medical Association.[8] She found that 75% of her sample was at or below the poor level of conditioning, with 33 of the 64 in poor shape. No one was in the excellent category and only three were very good. Based on these findings, Yiasemides concluded that aerobic fitness levels among female hospital personnel were surprisingly and unacceptably low.

In preparing material for this chapter, a survey of 35 head nurses and unit directors in Indiana was conducted to estimate the percentage of nurses who regularly exercise on a weekly basis. Estimates ranged from a low of 0.1% to a high of 30%, with a mean of 8.6%. These figures also suggest low fitness levels and participation rates among staff nurses.

Finally, Hobson and Walker are conducting an empirical analysis of fitness levels, participation rates, and perceptions among hospital nurses. Data have been collected from the staff in a 500-bed mid-western hospital. Six hundred questionnaires were distributed and 236 were completed and returned, for a response rate of 39.3%. Preliminary analyses indicate that 83 or 35.2% of the sample exercised at least three times/week on a regular basis. This is probably an inflated estimate of the actual percentage of all nurses in the hospital who are regularly engaged in fitness activities. The response rate was 39.3%, thus 60.7% did not complete the survey. In this situation, it would be reasonable to hypothesize that physically fit nurses would be more likely to respond to the survey than those who were not in shape. Therefore, the 35.2% figure is probably an overestimate of the percentage of total nurses exercising regularly. Unfortunately, the magnitude of this overestimation is unknown.

However, using the 35.2% figure, the results suggest that nearly two thirds of the nurses were not exercising at least three times each week. As a comparison, in the Gallup Survey mentioned earlier,[1] 63% of the women responding (both working and nonworking) were exercising regularly each week.

Given the meager empirical data available on nursing participation rates and fitness levels, the following tentative conclusions seem warranted: (1) compared to national figures, nurses seem to be exercising at rates lower than the general population, (2) most nurses are not currently involved in a regular fitness program, (3) fitness levels among most nurses are probably low, and (4) there is tremendous room for improvement in terms of fitness participation rates and levels among nurses.

The importance of fitness in nursing has been clearly established. Physically fit nurses can perform their duties more effectively and function better as appropriate fitness role models for others. In the next section, the research documenting the many personal and work-related benefits associated with fitness is reviewed. This accumulated evidence strongly argues for the vital necessity of fitness in nursing.

BENEFITS OF PHYSICAL FITNESS

A regular program of physical fitness can lead to benefits in two major categories: personal and work-related.

Personal Benefits

Substantial clinical and behavioral science research has documented the tremendous personal benefits of fitness in terms of both physiologic/physical and psychological factors. These benefits have been discussed and reviewed by several authors, including Brown,[6] Gurin and Harris,[1] Macnamara,[3] and Mirkin and Hoffman.[9] A list of the most significant physiologic/physical and psychological outcomes associated with increased levels of fitness is given in the box, Personal Benefits of Fitness.

Of particular importance to nurses, given the strenuous and stressful nature of their work are the following: (1) less susceptibility to illness, (2) increased energy level, (3) enhanced stamina, (4) improved muscle tone, power, strength, and endurance, and (5) relief of tension, stress, and frustration. In summary, the personal advantages linked to a regular fitness program are numerous and significant and can substantially improve the quality of one's life at work and in general.

Work-Related Benefits

Many studies are available examining the impact of fitness programs on work-related variables. This research has been summarized by several writers and includes estimates of the monetary value attributable to physically fit employees.[2,10-14]

Although the available literature consists of case studies and correlational research, and not the carefully controlled experimental designs necessary to establish direct causality, the findings are overwhelming in their consistency and support for the positive impact of fitness on a host of organizationally relevant

PERSONAL BENEFITS OF FITNESS

Physiologic/Physical
1. Reduced heart rate
2. Decreased blood pressure
3. Improved pulmonary and cardiovascular functioning
4. Reduced serum triglycerides, free fatty acids, and serum cholesterol
5. Decreased body fat
6. Improved sensory perception and motor responses
7. Decreased incidence of degenerative disease
8. Less susceptibility to illness
9. Retarded aging effects
10. Increased energy level
11. Enhanced stamina
12. Improved muscle tone, power, strength, and endurance
13. Increased coordination and range of motion
14. Better posture and flexibility
15. Improved sleep
16. Enhanced digestion
17. More attractive personal appearance

Psychological
1. Relief of tension, stress, and frustration
2. Improved mood
3. Increased life satisfaction
4. Enhanced ability to relax
5. Greater emotional stability and balance
6. Increased initiative and motivation
7. More fulfilling interpersonal relationships
8. Improved self-concept

---

variables. A list of the major work-related benefits associated with physical fitness programs is provided in the box, Work-Related Benefits of Fitness.

The factors in this box are essential determinants of organizational survival and success. Thus, improvements as a function of employee fitness levels can be invaluable in increasing efficiency and productivity and reducing costs. Some noteworthy examples taken from the aforementioned reviews will illustrate this point.

1. Employees at Battelle Institute Laboratories in Columbus, Ohio who regularly used the corporate fitness facilities averaged 2.8 days less absenteeism than those who did not. The

---

WORK-RELATED BENEFITS OF FITNESS

1. Higher job satisfaction
2. Reduced absenteeism and sick leave
3. Reduced turnover
4. Fewer errors and accidents
5. Reduced health care claims
6. Lower health care insurance premiums
7. Reduced premature death
8. Decreased life insurance premiums
9. Improved employee recruiting
10. Increased individual productivity
11. Higher overall organizational productivity

---

total savings from this reduction were calculated to be $150,000.00/year.

2. Xerox Corporation has estimated that the prevention of premature death or disability as a function of increased levels of physical fitness saves the company $600,000.00/year for each senior executive affected.

3. The National Institutes of Health has estimated that the average white-collar company can save $460,000.00 in annual medical costs for each 1,000 employees by promoting fitness and wellness.

4. Time Magazine reported that Berol Corporation reduced medical coverage premiums by $125,000.00/year due to the introduction of a corporate fitness program.[15] King Broadcasting Corporation was able to generate savings of $284,000.00 with a similar program.

5. Bowne, Russell, Morgan, Optenberg, and Clarke reported that a regional office of Prudential Insurance was able to generate an average reduction of $353.38 per person in major medical costs for physically fit employees as compared to the average operational expense of the corporate fitness facility of $120.60 per person.[16] Thus, the net savings per employee were $232.78.

The monetary benefits of physical fitness programs can be enormous. With the emphasis on cost containment in the health care industry, hospitals cannot afford to overlook the potential reward associated with corporate fitness programs. Nurses should act now and take a leading role in developing such programs and documenting their value.

MOTIVATING INDIVIDUAL FITNESS PARTICIPATION

The personal and work-related benefits of physical fitness are compelling. Consequently, concerted efforts should be focused on the problem of motivating high levels of employee participation. Although some individuals cannot exercise due to medical or physical problems, the vast majority are capable of exercising, if they *want to*. Hospital leaders can do a great deal to motivate their work force in this area. Organizations that are genuinely concerned about promoting employee fitness have a responsibility to establish and support on-site or in-house facilities. Such internal programs offer several advantages and can provide a cost-effective means of encouraging fitness participation.

Given that it is in an organization's own self-interest to promote employee fitness, the issue of motivating participation in corporate sponsored programs will be examined in more depth in this section.

The human motivation process can be conceptualized as consisting of three separate behavioral components that translate into three critical questions which must be addressed by any successful corporate fitness program (Table 12-1).

Motivation deals with the issue of what energizes or activates behavior. For example, why does an individual initially decide to begin physical training? Motivation is concerned with what gives behavior direction. For instance, from the many fitness options and programs available, why does a person choose one alterna-

Table 12-1. Three Behavioral Components of the Motivation Process and Applications to Fitness Programs

Behavior Components	*Application to Fitness Programs*
1. What initially *energizes* or *activates* behavior?	1. How can we motivate organizational members to want to become more physically fit and begin a fitness program?
2. What gives behavior *direction*?	2. How can we motivate organizational members to join the hospital sponsored fitness program?
3. What *sustains* behavior?	3. How can we motivate organizational members to continue to actively participate in the hospital fitness program over time?

tive over another and "move in that particular direction"? The third important component of motivation is what sustains behavior. For example, once a fitness program is started, why does an individual persist or continue participation in that program?

In order to most effectively encourage employee participation in corporate fitness programs, it is useful to view the motivational process as consisting of these three, separate and distinct components, each requiring different strategies on the part of management.

Although there can be an overlap or similarity in the methods that work well for each of the different components, approaches that are optimally suited to one component (*i.e.*, energizing) are not necessarily useful for either of the other two (directing or sustaining). Thus, in order to achieve maximum motivational effectiveness, it is recommended that corporate fitness proponents approach the participation issue by individually addressing each of the three components in the motivational process and developing customized strategies for use at each level.

What follows is a discussion of techniques for use in energizing, directing, and sustaining participation in corporate sponsored fitness programs. The specific strategies that are offered are not intended to represent a comprehensive or exhaustive listing of what might work. Rather, these suggestions are meant to provide examples of potentially useful approaches and further stimulate thinking and creativity in each area.

Energizing Behavior

The first component in the motivational process involves initially energizing or activating behavior; in other words, arousing the behavioral desire to begin a physical fitness program. Strategies designed to accomplish this objective generally focus on educating employees regarding the realistic costs and benefits involved, in an effort to overcome the tremendous obstacles — inertia and habit.

People commonly exhibit a strong tendency to resist major changes in their lives and this certainly applies to the changes associated with beginning a fitness program. Successfully overcoming this resistance and actually starting a program is contingent on an individual's belief that the perceived benefits will substantially outweigh the costs involved. Thus, a concerted effort should be made to effectively communicate comprehensive information concerning the advantages of being physically fit, as well as the disadvantages. This will allow employees to make accurate, informed participative decisions.

The dissemination of necessary information can be achieved in several ways. For instance, the active fitness involvement of top management is an excellent means of communicating support for fitness and its many benefits. Testimonials from top hospital managers can be effective in convincing employees of the advantages of fitness. In addition, fitness newsletters, brochures, and promotional films can be successfully used to convey critical information. Finally, a useful technique involves inviting employees, either individually or in small groups, to tour the corporate fitness center. An expert guide can introduce the program and its benefits and can also answer specific questions. In summary, various approaches are available to accomplish the objective of aggressively communicating the advantages of fitness to all employees.

In terms of the potential benefits associated with physical fitness, the favorable physiologic/physical improvements identified earlier should be emphasized. Most notably, these include such factors as (1) improved cardiovascular functioning, (2) lower blood pressure, (3) more efficient breathing, (4) better digestion, (5) weight loss, (6) improved sleep, (7) more energy, (8) more endurance, (9) greater muscle strength, (10) less frequent and less severe illness, (11) longer life expectancy, and (12) improved personal appearance. In addition, the positive psychological effects of physical conditioning should be noted: (1) enhanced mood, (2) improved self-concept, (3) greater satisfaction with work and life in general, and (4) increased ability to effectively handle stress. Taken together, the physiologic and psychological benefits of fitness are overwhelmingly positive and should be clearly and convincingly communicated to employees in an effort to initially energize or activate participation.

Although these physical and psychological advantages accrue directly to the individual, they also indirectly benefit the person's family, friends, and co-workers. This can form the basis of a powerful motivational message: "Don't just get in shape for yourself, do it for your loved ones and those you care about. By becoming more physically fit, one can become a better spouse, parent, friend or lover."

Another potentially important benefit of a corporate fitness program that is often overlooked is the opportunity for informal communication and interaction among employees from different levels and departments in the organization. The relationships that develop in the fitness center can lead to substantially improved organizational communication, coordination, conflict management, decision making, and overall functioning.

Finally, hospitals can create various additional benefits for employees who successfully begin and continue a fitness program. For example, some organizations pay employees a small amount (*e.g.*, 50 cents) for each mile run or its equivalent. Other companies provide extra vacation time to physically fit employees. Such corporate benefits can nicely complement the physiologic and psychological advantages of fitness and provide the necessary motivation to begin participation.

The "costs" associated with a fitness program should also be communicated to employees in order to dispel many common myths and fears and allow for more intelligent decisions concerning fitness participation. Many people, for example, are concerned about the potential health hazards associated with beginning a fitness program. To effectively address this important issue, a mandatory physical examination and medical approval should be required of all employees prior to their participation and qualified supervision (medical or exercise physiology background) available at all times. In this manner, fears of doing too much or doing the wrong exercises can be dispelled, as well as minimizing the possibility of injury.

Interestingly, many of the uncertainties, anxieties, and fears often associated with beginning a fitness program can be overcome by formally encouraging a buddy system approach. Using this format, employees are advised to begin working-out in pairs or small groups, thus sharing the experience and providing support for each other.

Another common misconception is that a fitness program will require an inordinate amount of time and energy. Success does require an individual commitment in terms of both time and effort. However, as the US Public Health Service has indicated, minimally acceptable levels of fitness can be maintained through a sustained 20-minute cardiovascular work-out three times each week. In fact, exercising more than three times weekly can have adverse effects in terms of both psychological burn-out and increased injury rates. While successfully beginning a fitness program requires a conscious decision to set aside time for exercising each week and respect for this commitment, lengthy, time-consuming, or daily work-outs are not necessary in structuring an effective program, especially in the initial stages.

In terms of progress in a fitness program, many have heard the popular expression "no pain, no gain," and believe that successful exercising is necessarily a painful experience. Nothing could be further from the truth or more counterproductive. Gradualism is the key to success!

An individual's exercise plan should match her capabilities and should be increased gradually as the person builds strength and endurance. A consistent commitment to three well-designed work-outs each week will result in slow, steady progress and increased strength and stamina. Dramatic improvements are difficult to attain and should not be the goal of an intelligent plan to begin a fitness program. Under no circumstances is it necessary or desirable to experience pain in the exercise process.

Finally, many people assume that athletic ability or coordination are essential for success in a fitness program. This assumption is both unfortunate and untrue. Physical fitness requires no special athletic ability and normal levels of coordination are more than adequate, as evidenced by the minimal requirements for running on a treadmill or riding a stationary cycle. Under the proper direction and supervision, an effective program can be tailored to match the unique athletic ability and coordination level of any individual.

The goal of energizing an employee's participation in a fitness program is to maximize the perceived benefits, while minimizing the perceived costs, thus providing a compelling rationale to overcome old habits, inertia, and resistance to the required behavioral changes. Ultimately, the objective is to begin a fitness program that will "fit-in" with one's life-style and be sustained over time. A knowledge of the advantages and disadvantages, rational planning, and a strong personal commitment are the keys to success in energizing or activating the necessary behavioral changes.

Directing Behavior

Once activation has occurred and an employee has made the commitment to try to become more physically fit, the next issue is what direction her behavior will take; that is, how will the person accomplish this task. A wide range of alternatives are possible, from a home work-out, to low-cost public gymnasiums, to expensive health clubs, to the corporate program. The challenge facing corporate fitness sponsors is essentially one of emphasizing and selling the comparative merits of their program over other available options. The return on in-house programs is gauged mainly on the degree of use and participation by employees. Expensive facilities that go unused are not generating an appropriate return.

Fortunately, in-house fitness programs often enjoy many objective advantages that should be communicated aggressively to employees. Most important among these are (1) proximity to the workplace, (2) convenience, (3) familiar surroundings and personnel, and (4) cost. Additional competitive advantages can be gained by offering (1) various modern, clean, well-maintained equipment in pleasant surroundings, (2) efficient shower and laundry facilities, (3) individualized attention, (4) both single sex and coed programs, (5) convenient systems for progress charting, and (6) professionally qualified, helpful, friendly, and attractive supervision and support staff.

Motivating employees in the direction of choosing the in-house program involves providing benefits not obtainable from other alternatives at a lower cost. Corporate programs must capitalize on their built-in advantages. They must pay special attention to the needs of individual employees in developing additional benefits, and they must vigorously disseminate this information throughout the organization.

Sustaining Behavior

Once an employee has initiated participation in a corporate fitness program, the critical issue becomes how to sustain that behavior. The importance of this issue is emphasized by the fact that virtually everyone has started a fitness program at some point in their lives, but few continue it. The numerous positive benefits of fitness for the individual and organization are only made possible through a program of sustained physical activity. Viewed in this manner, the most important measure of success is the sustainability of fitness efforts. An employee should be encouraged to develop a personalized program that matches her life-style and can be continued indefinitely. Brown has stressed the importance of this fact in nursing.[6] This ultimate objective of sustainability should be emphasized constantly to all participants.

Several potentially useful strategies in motivating continued participation are available to fitness program managers. For example, a common problem causing early termination involves the false expectation of rapid progress in terms of strength, bulk, definition, endurance, or weight loss. Employees should receive comprehensive information concerning the physiologic process underlying physical fitness, which emphasizes the gradual nature of these changes. Dramatic improvements are highly unlikely. False hopes and expectations can be successfully countered in this manner, thus helping to keep people realistically involved in their fitness effort. Participants can expect slow, but steady physiologic progress to result from conscientious work-outs three times each week.

With this in mind, one excellent technique to motivate sustained participation is to provide employees with a convenient and systematic method for charting their progress in terms of such factors as (1) the number of repetitions of each exercise, (2) the length of each exercise, (3) the amount of weight used, and (4) bodily changes in heart rate, blood pressure, and weight. This type of feedback information allows participants to document their own progress and observe the slow steady nature of the improvements that occur. Over a 6-month period, the improvements can be substantial and rewarding.

Another related problem that confronts individuals who have participated over a period of time is the eventual encounter with a progress plateau. In the initial stages of any fitness program, progress is slow but steady, predictable, and inevitable with concerted effort. This progress can serve as a powerful reinforcer and reward for the participant. However, eventually most people reach a plateau, from which further progress is difficult and slow in developing.

Some plateaus are natural characteristics of the fitness process and should be communicated to all participants. The demotivating, discouraging impact of progress plateaus, which can often lead to the termination of participants from the program, can be effectively dealt with by educating employees in advance and realistically structuring their expectations.

Maintaining interest and active participation in a corporate fitness program can be facilitated by providing various pieces of equipment and activities. There are countless ways in which fitness can be achieved and many different types of exercises to develop specific muscle groups, including nautilus equipment, weight training, dance – aerobics, swimming, cycling, and jogging.

A variety of activities and exercises can help stimulate the interest of the participants and can encourage continued commitment. Corporate fitness directors should strive to develop as many different programs and activities as possible in order to prevent employees from being victimized by a boring fitness routine and perhaps leaving the program.

The "buddy system," mentioned earlier as a means of overcoming the initial anxiety often associated with starting a fitness program, can also function effectively to encourage continued participation. Peer involvement and social support can combine to motivate employees, who might otherwise have left, to continue their fitness efforts. Thus, corporate program managers should strongly recommend the participation of pairs or small groups of employees as a powerful way to motivate continued attendance.

A commonly cited reason for stopping a fitness program arises when a busy executive is forced to be out of town frequently or for a long time. Such interruptions can be discouraging and can lead to decisions to stop participating. Fitness program managers should therefore develop convenient travel work-outs that could be done in the privacy of one's hotel room and might include for example, various calisthenics and running in place. Travel work-outs could be tailored specifically to an individual's level of fitness by a staff exercise physiologist prior to departure.

Given the rapid loss of strength and endurance experienced during prolonged lay-offs, the goal of the travel work-out would be to maintain one's basic conditioning until regular participation could resume. This would help employees sustain their interest, commitment, and level of fitness during periods away from the corporate facility.

In order to sustain high rates of employee participation, the fitness facility staff must be knowledgeable, competent, helpful, and friendly. They must be trained thoroughly in both the physiologic and psychological aspects of the fitness process. In addition, they must be sensitive to individual differences and aware of their important roles as motivators in providing encouragement and support. Finally, excellent staff interpersonal skills can help make the fitness process a more enjoyable, rewarding experience, thereby facilitating continued employee participation.

As mentioned earlier, the ultimate goal of any fitness program is sustaining participation over time. Individual employees need to be convinced that the benefits of fitness occur only with continued participation. Their objective should be to develop a fitness routine that can be continued throughout their lives. Fitness program managers can imaginatively use many of the aforementioned strategies to assist employees in sustaining their fitness participation.

This section has presented a conceptual model of the motivational process consisting of three separate components (energizing, directing, and sustaining) and related it directly to the issue of employee fitness participation rates. Different strategies are required to effectively motivate individuals at each stage in the process and several potentially useful techniques are presented. This information will hopefully assist proponents of corporate fitness programs in better motivating employee participation.

ACTION PLAN FOR NURSING LEADERS

In terms of promoting physical fitness, nursing leaders have special responsibilities in three major areas. First, nurse leaders should demonstrate their commitment to fitness by following a rigorous personal program. Managers can significantly enhance their own productivity, satisfaction, and health by engaging in regular fitness activities. Nursing leaders must capitalize on this information and maximize their own performance.

Furthermore, nurse leaders must provide appropriate role models for their staff, patients, and the general public. Physically fit nursing leaders will be infinitely more effective in promoting fitness among others. The message is simple: "practice what you preach." Nursing leaders can have a significant positive impact on the fitness habits of their staff, patients, and the public by their actions and attitudes.

Given the overwhelming personal and work-related benefits of fitness, nursing leaders have a responsibility to aggressively pursue the establishment and support of hospital fitness programs.[7,8] Regrettably, Yiasemides has observed that employee fitness programs are rarely found in hospitals. If institutions are serious about physical fitness, they must develop organization-wide programs and promote participation. Nurses are ideally suited to take a lead role in this process.

Success in the operation of a hospital-wide program requires the following elements: (1) top management support and participation, (2) convenient on-site or in-house facilities, (3) paid time-off to exercise three times each week, and (4) rewards and incentives to encourage sustained participation and high levels of fitness.[15] The costs of such a comprehensive approach are not trivial; however, the benefits far outweigh these costs.

Improved levels of physical fitness will help nurses and other hospital employees be healthier, less stressed, and enjoy their lives more. In addition, job performance will improve and personnel costs will decrease significantly. Given the labor intensive nature of the hospital business, any strategy to improve employee health and productivity will result in substantial savings. Again, nurses should take a leadership role in disseminating this information and acting on it.

By virtue of education, training, and work experience, the nurse is uniquely positioned to advocate and promote fitness to patients, businesses, and to the public. A well informed, enthusiastic, physically fit nurse can function as an outstanding, credible spokesperson and catalyst for fitness programs. Nursing leaders have a special responsibility to encourage and support the involvement of nurses in developing fitness awareness and motivating higher participation rates in all segments of the population.

Many hospitals are expanding their services by enlisting nurses to formulate and operate fitness/wellness centers. Many nurse entrepreneurs have also seized the opportunity provided by the prevailing interest in fitness in the United States and they have developed thriving businesses offering fitness/wellness services themselves.

Fitness is thus important in nursing for several reasons. Success in promoting fitness and reaping the many associated benefits will depend largely on the efforts of nursing leaders, who must rise to the occasion and meet the challenge.

SUMMARY AND CONCLUSIONS

1. Interest in fitness, health, and wellness in the United States has increased dramatically in all segments of the population, including businesses and corporations.

2. Within nursing, fitness is important for two major reasons: (a) the job of nurses is physically demanding and requires a high level of fitness in order to be effective and (b) nurses have a special responsibility as role models and leaders in promoting health and fitness.

3. Empirical research addressing fitness participation rates and levels among nurses is poor. However, based on the available evidence, the following conclusions seem warranted: (a) compared to national statistics, nurses seem to be exercising at rates lower than the general population, (b) most nurses are not involved in a regular fitness program, (c) fitness levels among most nurses are probably low, and (d) there is tremendous room for improvement in terms of fitness participation rates and levels.

4. The personal benefits of fitness consist of many important physiologic/physical and psychological factors.

5. Fitness results in several significant work-related benefits, and the monetary savings associated with these factors can be substantial.

6. The process of motivating participation in fitness activities consists of three components: energizing behavior, directing behavior, and sustaining behavior. Different specific strategies should be used with each one to maximize overall motivation.

7. In terms of promoting fitness, nursing leaders have special responsibilities in three major areas: (a) to engage in regular exercise programs in order to maximize personal productivity and health and function as an appropriate role model for staff members and others, (b) to vigorously promote effective hospital-wide fitness programs, and (c) to encourage nurses to act as spokespersons and catalysts in promoting fitness programs of patients, businesses, and the public.

Questions for Reflection and Discussion

1. Why has physical fitness become so popular in the United States?

2. Why is physical fitness so important in the nursing profession?

3. What are the major personal benefits—both physiologic and psychological—associated with physical fitness? Which of these are more important in the nursing profession?

4. What are the major work-related outcomes associated with physically fit employees?

5. Is a physically fit nurse a more cost-effective and productive nurse? Support your response and give examples.

6. Why do many nurses fail to participate regularly in physical fitness activities?

7. How can an understanding of the three components in the individual motivational process help a manager to encourage more nurses to engage regularly in physical fitness activities?

8. What can be done to sustain participation in fitness programs?

9. What special responsibilities do nursing leaders have in promoting fitness?

10. Briefly develop and describe an ideal hospital program designed to maximize fitness participation among nurses.

REFERENCES

1. Gurin J, Harris TG: Exclusive Gallup Survey: The happy health confidents. Am Health VI(2): 53–57, 1987
2. Higdon H: Working out at work. The Runner 9(4): 26–31, 1987
3. Macnamara EL: Fitting nursing into fitness. J Canad Nurse 176(4): 33–35, 1980
4. Millen HM: Physically fit for nursing. Am J Nurs 70(3): 520–523, 1970
5. Race GA: Oh my aching . . . J Pract Nurs 27(2): 26, 40, 1979
6. Brown BS: Fitting fitness into your life. Nurs Economics 1: 93–96, 1983
7. Rimer B, Glassman B: The fitness revolution: Will nurses sit this one out? Nurs Econ 1: 84–89, 144, 1983
8. Yiasemides E: Aerobic fitness: How do hospital personnel measure up? Occup Health Nurs 30(3): 24–28, 1982
9. Mirkin G, Hoffman M: The Sports Medicine Book. New York, Little Brown, 1978
10. Donoghue S: The correlation between physical fitness, absenteeism, and work performance. Canad J Public Health 68: 201–203, 1977
11. Hoffman JJ, Hobson CJ: Physical fitness and employees effectiveness. Personal Administrator April 1984, pp 101–113, 126
12. Pelfrey S, Hobson CJ: Keeping employees physically fit can be cost efficient. Man Accounting LXV(12): 39–43, 1987
13. Pyle RL: Performance measures for a corporate fitness program. Hum Res Man 18: 26–30, 1979
14. Smith KJ, Haight GT, Everly GS, Jr.: Evaluating corporate wellness investments. The Internal Auditor Feb, 1986, pp 28–34
15. Health and Fitness—Giving Goodies to the Good. Time Magazine Nov 8, 1985, p 98
16. Bowne DW, Russell ML, Morgan JL et al: Reduced disability and health care costs in an industrial fitness program. J Occup Med 26(11): 809, 816, 1984

13
Nursing at a Crossroads

THE PURPOSE of this chapter is to describe the professional nurse, the professional practice, the consumer, and the setting or environment during the transition of the health care system into the 21st century.

Nursing as a process involves someone diagnosing and treating human responses to an actual or potential health problem.[1] The components at all times should include a nurse (someone), a practice (responding to an actual or potential health problem), a consumer (someone), and a setting (somewhere). The future of both nursing and health care is contingent on varied interacting elements that effect trends in society, economic conditions, and human values.[2]

Predicting the future setting for health care delivery is no less difficult than predicting the future for the other three components in the nursing process. All writers agree that it will differ greatly from the present health care setting.

SOCIETAL CHANGES

Society itself will change dramatically and these changes will greatly influence health care and nursing. Nurses should be aware of the anticipated changes in order to take advantage of the opportunities presented. For example, in Naisbitt's popular book *Megatrends*,[3] ten new directions transforming our lives are expounded on. They include the following:

1. Move to an information society from an industrial society
2. Beginning of a high tech society with a compensatory human response of high touch
3. Operation of a global economy versus one that is independent in each country
4. Move to long term planning from short term planning
5. Decentralization of the country
6. Shift to more self-reliance in all phases of our existence from institutional dependence
7. Era of participatory democracy through immediate shared news in place of a representative democracy
8. Development of an informal networking process instead of formal hierarchies
9. Shift in the population in America to the South and West from the North and East
10. Outbreak of a multiple-option society from a restricted either/or one of few personal options (pp 1–2).[3]

HEALTH CARE DELIVERY SYSTEM

One of the long-held and widely accepted views of the health care delivery setting is that it will be dominated by relatively few corporations.[4] This view, however, has been challenged by health care policy experts participating in an American Hospital Association teleconference entitled, *The CEO Challenge: Payment, Finance, and Delivery.* They dismissed the earlier predictions that seven or eight large corporations would control the delivery of health care.[5] Thomas First, M.D., Chairman and Chief Executive Officer of Hospital Corporation of America, stated that he believed all hospitals would have to associate with other providers in order to survive.[5] What form these alliances would take and how close the association or how centralized the control would be was unclear.

Jeff Goldsmith, Ph.D. (President of Health Futures Inc., and National Technical Advisor of Ernest and Whinney), offered his opinion on why a few large corporations would not dominate the field.[6] Health care is not a commodity and, therefore, the providers do not have the type of pressure or incentives that cause industries to merge. Survival in the health care field is not guaranteed by merger. Market positions are not automatically improved by increasing size or adding capital. The strategic choices that a hospital makes will determine its future success. A hospital with good cost controls, a first-rate medical staff, and a strong market base will probably be able to survive.[5]

In this competitive environment nursing will play a key role in marketing the hospital's services to its constituency. There is an alarming tendency on the part of some managers to characterize hospitals as delivering a product. Products are manufactured or produced and they represent consistency. Products are usually inanimate in that, when purchased or consumed, there is usually nothing the seller can do to change them. Services, on the other hand, are performed; they are not produced. Services are perceived as being highly personal and tied closely to the environment: they depend on the performance of an individual or groups of individuals and on the ambiance of the setting.[6] A hospital's future survival will depend on its ability to retain or enhance its share of market, which in turn will depend on the delivery of nursing services.

Regardless of whether the health care delivery system is dominated by some large corporations (either for profit or not-for-profit) or by many medium-sized organizations, some form of association among providers will be the mode of operation.

The hospital in its present form will no longer exist. It will be replaced by a system of clinics, surgicenters, emergicenters, birthing centers, and other types of ambulatory out-patient settings.

The diagnostic related group (DRG) system forced providers to look at the use of hospitals from a different perspective. The result has been fewer admissions and patients spending a shorter time in hospital. This trend will continue until the inpatient level of acuity is comparable to that in the present intensive care units. A patient's length of stay in the hospital will not be beyond his need for the life-saving technology and clinical expertise available only in the hospital setting. An extended care facility or the home will be the site of recovery. Only medically unstable patients will remain in the hospital. These patients, once stabilized, will move on to another setting.[7]

Advances in medical technology have made it possible in the community hospital to perform procedures on a routine basis that were done only in research centers or were only in the initial stages 20 years ago. However, as we move into the 21st century the highly visible advances such as organ transplants and artificial organs may not have the most lasting effects on the health care system. Rather, advances in diagnostic imaging and improved clinical information systems, combined with progress in anesthesia and less invasive surgical procedures, may have a more profound effect on the future of health care delivery.[6]

INFORMATION AGE

Many sophisticated forms of communication, such as television and computers, have affected our lives significantly in the last 35 years. The new technology involves not only more software and hardware but also innovative ways of thinking and doing. This revolution in communications, with its inherent dependence on advances in technology, has had an increasing impact on the decisions of the health provider about resources, regarding whether to acquire new technology, to cooperate with other agencies, or to forfeit potential advances in health care.[8]

TELEMATICS

Information becomes even more copious, intricate, and highly specific as society moves into the 21st century. New methods of coping with this information explosion have been developed. *Telematics* is the term for this new technology. Milio states,

> "It allows *interaction* between machines and people and produces *synergies* (multiple effects) among machines and the communications systems that bind video, computers, and satellites. Specifically, telematics consists of the hardware and software of telecommunications technologies (*e.g.*, cable, satellite, digital telephone, and direct broadcast television), computers, and video technologies (*e.g.*, video recorders, videodiscs) plus their combinations into new networks (*e.g.*, multiple distribution services, low power TV,

mobile telephone systems), services (*e.g.*, videotex and pay TV), and industries (*e.g.*, electronic mail, publishing, and entertainment), all made possible by low unit costs of microcomputers and laser and optical fiber advances" (p 39).[9]

Forecasters such as Lutz,[10] Turner,[11] Dawson,[12] Bezold,[13] Carlson,[14] and Milio[9] are foreseeing the use of telematics in the future of health care. A sample of what will be possible technologically includes (1) the uniting and distribution of all sources of data on patients and expert knowledge into a medical information systems, (2) the enhancement and increased effectiveness of laboratory tests through computers, (3) the establishment of regional information centers for practitioners, (4) the use of computer-assisted instruction in self-learning continuing education, (5) the linkage of environmental and epidemiologic data on a systemwide basis that will aid in the reduction of infectious diseases, (6) an aggregate national data pool connecting knowledge about the patient with drug and other therapy preventing adverse affects and decreasing law suits, (7) computer applied standards that will abate ethical dilemmas regarding who will receive treatment, (8) new distinctions within health professionals involving the "mappers" (the creators of the computer artificial intelligence that help solve diagnostic and therapeutic problems for the nonexpert clinical computer user) and the practitioners who use this system and provide raw data feedback in order to continuously upgrade it, (9) practitioners will be able to monitor patients from a distance by implanted patient sensors, and individuals will be knowledgeable of these techniques and monitor their own health status at home ("hospital-on-the-wrist"), a microchip with a person's health history will be mounted on a type of credit card ("Smart Card Health Record") allowing for operative linkages among providers of health care, and (10) generalized and personalized computer programs and videodiscs for home use on topics such as diet, exercise, stress reduction, psychotherapy, and prescribed and over-the-counter drugs.

The patients/clients in the 21st century will be connected to either physicians' offices, HMOs, clinics, hospitals, or various types of "centers" by a system of telematics that will make it possible for the home or the residential community to return as the primary site of clinical care. This situation is similar to the one at the start of the 20th century.[6]

HEALTHY LIFE-STYLES FOR CONSUMERS

As the health system focus moves from a illness – wellness orientation through a wellness – illness transitional period to a less costly health prescriptive mode,[15] consumers will assume more responsibility for their own health and the health of members of their families. A great emphasis will continue to be placed on proper nutrition and physical fitness in maintaining a healthy body. Individuals and families will be committed to a well balanced nutritious diet, exercise program, stress reduction techniques, health-promoting life-styles that include a freedom from smoking environment, and control of risks such as abuse of drugs and alcohol and the use of seat belts.

Healthy life-styles will become the way of life for the average American. Individuals, through their own self-awareness or through peer pressure will realize this is the least costly way to live.

Graying of America

In 1980, more than 1% of the population, over two million Americans, was more than 85 years old. This category of individuals is growing faster than any other group. They are referred to as the old old, the oldest old, or the extreme aged. In 2020, there will be over 7 million or 2.5% in this population group.[16]

During the 20th century the average life expectancy has increased from under 50 years to over 70 years. Another major trend is the baby boomers' generation: 76.4 million persons were born from 1946 to 1964. An analogy to the impact of this group would be to watch the digestion process of a boa constrictor that has swallowed a whole small animal. First the schools felt the impact, next came the job market. As this generation ages, pension plans, social security, medical care will be affected. The population aged 65 years and older will total 50 million retirees by 2030 (two times greater than in the early 1980s).[16]

After age 75, sickness and mortality rates accelerate, which have an impact on the development of health and social services. Butler states, "Between 1980 and 2020, the 75-and-over population with activity limitations due to chronic conditions will increase 2.5 times, to 10.7 million. The number of short-stay hospitalizations will rise to 104.6 million days from 45.8 million. Instead of 1.1 million in nursing homes, there will be 2.7 million. The number of physician visits will double. Personal expenditure for health care will more than double for the aged, while it rises by 50 percent for the entire U.S. population. Nursing home expenditures will be in the forefront".[16]

Chronically Ill

Throughout the life cycle, from the very young to the elderly, individuals with chronic illnesses have special needs. Over the years all of the advanced technology and pharmaceutical innovations have changed the course of disease and the time of death.

In 1980, excluding the mentally ill or retarded, an estimated 3,823,098 people in the United States were categorized as chronically ill or disabled. Of that group, 7.6% were between 17 and 64 years of age. Even though the health care needs of adults and children with chronic illnesses are different, they both have a need for a case manager, someone who has the responsibility for health maintenance, coordinating necessary services, and enhancing the quality of life. Hospitals and communities are also linked by the chronically ill of all ages. As a group and at great costs they regularly use the service and spend time in both hospitals and the primary care sector.[17]

Acutely Ill

From 1983 to 1986 there was a dramatic 20% increase in inpatient acuity. During that same time the availability of hospital beds for the acutely ill dropped from 1250/100,000 of population to 1000/100,000. By 1995, the number of beds necessary for this type of patient will stabilize at about 450/100,000 of population. Curtin makes the assumption that, "Acuity rates will continue to rise as numbers of beds fall until, by 1995, anyone admitted to a short-term acute care hospital would have been placed in an intensive care unit in 1982" (p 7).[18]

NURSING IN THE 21ST CENTURY

The nurse in the 21st century has to be exceptionally astute in perceiving alternatives and seeking innovative methods to resolve issues. This is the only way their knowledge, ability, and level of satisfaction will remain dynamic, credible, and at a high level of excellence.

The new era in health care delivery provides several alternatives for nurses to claim new roles that will be essential for both the public they serve and for the nursing profession. Some of these new opportunities are found in acute care hospitals where nurses have previously been the brunt of considerable scrutiny.[17]

Future Leadership — Personal and Professional Assets

Sovie is straightforward in her description of the stormy times the health-care industry is facing with the subsequent erosion and disappearance of traditional practices. There is a critical need for effective leadership during the creation of new clinical practices and patterns.[19]

The personal and professional assets of the future nurse manager necessary for inclusion in the wider problem solving process are outlined by Porter–O'Grady.[15] These include the following:

1. Well internalized sense of self in order to promote excellent relationships with others

2. Relational and problem solving skills that provide nursing power to decide complex problems in the environment

3. Collaborative, respective relationship with all health professionals in joint problem solving

4. Clear understanding of nursing roles and responsibilities of professional practice for all health professionals including the nurse

5. Broad understanding of health care issues and "an awareness of policy, governance, economic, and social issues related to the delivery of health care services" (p 203).[15]

The effective nurse leader will be involved in both economic and health care decisions that affect the delivery of services. Professional nurses will have in-depth knowledge of the delivery system. Porter–O'Grady describes the role transition into the 21st century of the nurse, which includes role expectations, accountabilities, and nursing care functions (Fig. 13-1).[15]

The following shift in role responsibility/accountability, and function of professional nursing will occur during the transition into the 21st century (Fig. 13-1).

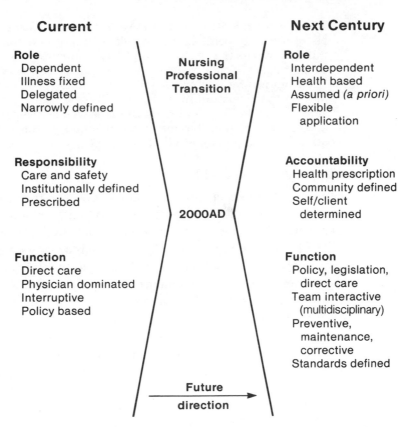

FIGURE 13-1. *Role transition into the 21st century. (Porter–O'Grady T: Creative Nursing Administration: Participative Management into the 21st Century. Reprinted with permission of Aspen Publishers, Inc., Rockville, MD. © 1986)*

Types of Role

1. The role will change from a dependent to an interdependent one. The key to the interdependent role is collaboration among the nurse, consumer, physician, and all other health professionals instead of a dependent role on the physician.

2. The role will be health-based instead of illness fixed. Emphasis will be on the prevention of illness through promotion of health. Society will incorporate this change in its economic and social systems of health care delivery.

3. As powerful professionals, nurses will assume new roles instead of waiting for them to be delegated by the physician and others. Such a role would be shaping the corporate culture.[19]

4.   The nurse's role will need to have a flexible application *vs* being narrowly defined. There will be many new roles for nurses both in the hospitals and the community. Sovie is suggesting this change when she describes the need for, "new norms for many settings — the nurse as a valued partner, participating in decisions affecting the delivery of care and the business of organization as well as the nurse as a care giver, responsible for providing quality, compassionate care to patients and families" (p 17).[19]

Responsibility and Accountability

The responsibility of the professional nurse will shift from that of a narrow care and safety focus to accountability of a broader role in determining the health prescription of the client/patient.

This responsibility will be defined not only from an institutional perspective but will also include the accountability of the nurse defined from a community perspective. Professional nurses will be identified as vital emissaries of the institution. According to Hafer and Joiner,[20] "Since the nurse is the most visible health-care professional to both the patient and the patient's family, the nurse has a substantial impact on the patient's image of the hospital, the type of care being received, and the word-of-mouth image created by the patient's family throughout the community" (p 26).[20] Professional nurses will be the recognized binding force of the health care system.

From the current method of prescribed nursing responsibilities, professional nurses will move to a self/client determined accountability. The future role of nursing will emerge from the needs of the clientele, who ideally will enter the total system of health care through a mechanism of health promotion and health maintenance.

Function

The professional nursing function of direct care will be broadened to include policy, legislation, and direct care. Professional nurses will become partners with administrators and physicians in the business of health care. As such, they will play a key role in establishing policy, in influencing legislation, and in providing direct care.

There will be a shift from physician-dominated to multidisciplinary team interactive function. In this respect the professional nurse will frequently be in control with regard to the health plan for the client/patient.

The interruptive nature of health care will switch to a preventive, maintenance, corrective care. This direction of total health care will be a major function of professional nurses because of their comprehensive knowledge of the delivery system.

Policy-based function of professional nursing will change to standards defined. A framework such as is provided by the American Nurses' Association Standards of Practice and Social Policy Statement gave professional norms and direction to the nurse, which is consistent nationally as compared to narrowly focused institutional policies. The ownership is on the professional nurse through standards instead of the institution through its policies. "The new viewpoint is that professional nurses offer a specified service to the institution rather than that the facility owns its framework for nursing."[15]

PROFESSIONAL PRACTICE

Nursing practice in the 21st century will be intimate, compassionate, empathetic, and professional.

Knowledge Exclusive in Nature

A new script for education must be written in order to prepare professional nurses for the information age. "The knowledge base of practice will be well-delineated and unique in that its use will enable the practitioner to offer services for which there is no substitution. A profession reflects the acquisition of knowledge and skills by its members that no other group possesses. There is no substitution for the professional. The knowledge of nursing must be exclusive in nature" (p 119).[21]

One of the most important factors assuring a well prepared professional nurse in the future will be the requirement of the baccalaureate degree in nursing as the minimal requirement for entry into the profession. The future undergraduate curriculum will include, in addition to clinical content, the business of health care, including health care economics, cost control, cost accounting, cost-effective strategies, management of human resources, systems management, institutional and peer governance, and power, politics, and policy making. All professional nurses, whether they serve as case managers or corporate executives, must have a high degree of knowledge of the complexities of the health delivery system both internal and external to their practice.[15,19]

Graduate and postgraduate program offerings will be comprehensive in the areas of economics and policy. Diers states, "There are three general content areas in policy: money, power, and history. In each case, there are bodies of knowledge available, such as economics, finance, political science, large and small group behavior, and authority relationships and there are well-described case reports of the influences of power and money on health care" (p 45).[22]

Nurses in advanced practice will need knowledge bases that will provide a variety of interpretations for the behaviors they will encounter. "They need to know probability reasoning; how to judge the likelihood of a prediction, given the findings from observation or examination, and the slipperiness of the known 'facts'" . . . "Clinical judgment is best taught from a research base, the research literature. Students learn probability theory from assembling 'known' data, finding gaps in knowledge, and making predictions of likely outcome."[22] These professional nurses will have the vision and knowledge to forecast trends and issues of the health care delivery system including those that will have an economic impact.

Education is a lifelong process. In addition to education through formal academic programs, short, intensive continuing education offerings, such as were described in Chapter 2, are necessary to promote cost-effective nursing practice.

Automated Information System

Since the early 1980s because of reimbursement policies, hospital administrators have been energetically evaluating the cost-effectiveness of automated information systems. These systems were designed primarily to capture the charges for each patient and had little to do with the patient's care. In the latter half of the decade nursing executives began to seriously analyze their needs for a system capable of providing clinical and management data.[23] Such systems offer the possibility of monitoring and improving the patient care process in much the same way as statistical process control (SPC) techniques have been used in business and industry to enhance productivity.[24]

As we move into the decade of the nineties, Mowry and Korpman describe the ideal hospital information system.[23]

> The ideal hospital information system designed to support the business of health care in today's marketplace is an integrated system that has data entry and data retrieval devices located at the patient's bedside and at every work station in the ancillary departments throughout the hospital. The ideal system will be centered around a single hospital-wide database built through the use of tables and a software support system that allows users to change the database using simple tools. Nurses, physicians, and other clinicians will have the flexibility of producing database and screen format changes to keep pace with their dynamic practice patterns and to define the data-filtering criteria that will make the system maximally useful to each category of provider.
>
> Additionally, the system will be highly menu driven for speed and simplicity of data entry, standardization of documentation, and facilitation of statistical analysis in research studies. To meet the described requirements, the entire medical record will be kept on-line indefinitely" (pp 11–12).[23]

Some of the important advantages of such a system follow:

1. Nursing time on clerical functions is significantly reduced.
2. Documentation has increased quality.
3. Interdepartmental communications are accurate and enhanced.
4. Expensive mistakes of omission and duplication are abolished.
5. Patient care scheduling is optimal by including both nursing and physician prescriptions.
6. Interventions to patient outcomes are easily tracked.
7. Quality assurance programs (on-line) are better, using system-provided audit trails.
8. Research capacities in management are far-ranging.
9. Use of nursing assessments and care plans through on-line menus is enhanced.
10. Suggestive staffing patterns in relation to patient acuity are automatically calculated.
11. Resources, both personnel and supplies, can be directly limited by DRG and patient.
12. The inventory of supplies can be monitored and reordered as they are used.
13. All types of data and reports can be generated as needed.

14. The evaluation of productivity outcomes will be expedited.

15. On-line, provider-specified data are available for easy and objective support of departmental standards, clinical ladders, and performance evaluations.

16. Computer-assisted instruction for both the patient and health care provider can be readily available to meet a variety of educational needs, as well as a built in evaluation component of the effectiveness of the program.[23]

As conceptualized and described in Chapter 2, the professional nurse should be in the key, pivotal role of controlling costs. A thorough understanding and involvement in the automated information system of hospitals will be essential in future decades for professional nurses to assume this powerful role.

Collaborative Practice

In a restrictive economic environment, "turf issues" between health professionals are likely to develop if a collaborative interdisciplinary team approach does not exist. The collaborative practice model of the future must differ greatly from the traditional model if cost-effective care is a reality. It represents an interdependent cooperative effort between the patient/client and members of the health care team *vs* authority flowing downward from the physician through the professional nurse, ancillary personnel, to the patient.[25]

A common philosophy of care and mutually established goals is important for collaborative practice. This is evident to all individuals concerned when a collaborative practice model exists. Patient outcomes are improved through coordination of discharge planning, a thorough understanding and demonstration of effective communications among team members, and an efficient and effective support service. Furthermore, critical to cost-effective collaborative practice is that health care executives are members of the team. Simms and associates state, "To be successful, this innovation requires both effort and commitment, but the benefits are enormous for patients, professionals, and cost containment" (p 37).[26]

Professionalism and competence are important for successful collaborative practice. Each health team member must not only know her roles and abilities but those of all of the team members.

"Team players must also understand and appreciate one another's value. Collaborative practice does not involve the substitution of labor, but rather the efficient utilization of personnel in roles they are prepared to assume" (p 44).[26]

Education for the nurse on this multidisciplinary team must be at the professional level. Skills will be needed in such areas as management, clinical practice, interpersonal relations, and group dynamics. They must be included in formal academic programs and periodically updated and enhanced through continuing education. "Varied educational and competency levels and resistance to added responsibility have hampered the development of collaborative practice" (p 44).[26]

Perrin states, "When nurses and physicians are asked what is the basis of collaboration, three things are always mentioned: Communication, competency, and trust. Inadequacies of either profession in preparation and continuing development are not conducive to success in joint practice. These are pivotal evaluation factors" (pp 557–560).[27]

Flexibility is a key factor of the collaborative practice model because it can be used in all areas of practice. The components may change, that is, the individuals, the organization and setting, but the major theme, providing quality care, remains the same. Comprehensive care is provided within this framework in a qualitative manner, costs are controlled, and practitioners feel professionally satisfied because their skills and expertise are used appropriately. Professional nurses must endeavor to educate the nurses of the future, physicians, and all health professionals in the concept of this model in order to ensure that it forms the foundation of the health care delivery system of the future.

Reimbursement for Professional Practice

Aydelotte[21] projects the total health system of the 21st century as including four branches where nurses will practice: (1) health promotion and maintenance, (2) dramatic episodic care, (3) chronic disease management, and (4) care of the elderly, frail, and dying. Within these branches, four types of roles will evolve for professional nurses: (1) direct care giver, (2) case manager, (3) executive, and (4) researcher.

The question of how the professional nurse will be renumerated is critical to the future of nursing. Curtin states, "The fee-for-service system is dead, although it will take a few years to put the nails in the coffin. However, by 2000 AD, 98 percent of reimbursement for health services will be by contract, capitation or medical condition" (p 8).[18] Payment for professional nursing practice will be an integral part of this reimbursement system.

Nursing services will be provided through various employment arrangements, for example: (1) nurses may form professional corporations that will then contract as a group to provide nursing services to schools, businesses, hospices, intensive care units, (2) there may be nurse specialty practice groups that then, on an individual basis, contract with clients to provide special services, (3) there may be nurses who practice as individuals and contract to provide highly specialized nursing service on an individual basis as they provide consultation to other nurses and professionals, and (4) there will be traditional employment in the health care system that will be mainly acute care nursing.[21]

Key to the payment in the acute care arrangement is that the nursing operations are designed as a profit center instead of a cost center. As a profit center, managers are responsible for both costs and revenues. The responsibility for deficits and profits is also assumed. This mechanism must exist at all levels of nursing operations in order to be successful. The efficiency, effectiveness, and efficacy of the nursing department will be evaluated on the basis of the profit it makes.[29]

Entrepreneurial/Intrapreneurial Behaviors

Nursing will be identified increasingly as a business, and nurses will need to develop a more business-like managerial attitude toward practice. Nurses must become entrepreneurs. An entrepreneur is one who assumes the risk and management of business. For nurses who work in hospitals the more correct term would be *intrapreneurs*. Intrapreneurs exhibit entrepreneurial behaviors within an organization. Nursing is a service business and, if nurse intrapreneurs are to compete successfully, it will be because they care more about patients and because they market this fact.

Autonomy is a key characteristic of both professionals and of entrepreneurs/intrapreneurs. A system that promotes entrepreneurship makes it possible to be entrepreneutral but not self-employed. Corporate management will be a vital support system for each head nurse/manager, a channel to share ideas, communicate experiences, anticipate potential results, and solve problems. A prime motivator for entrepreneurs to do their best is pride in their work, even though the work is hard. As we move into the 21st century, each nurse must have a need for achievement and a commitment to quality cost-effective care.

CONCLUSIONS

Research in the clinical setting will increase and will be directed toward assisting with documentation that nursing makes a difference. The difference will be evident in a reduction of the hospital stay, the importance of the nursing diagnosis, quality assurance, patient education, and planning for the patient's discharge.

Nurses will not only face the challenge of prospective payment, but nurses will constitute a major force in shaping the delivery of health care in the 21st century.

Questions for Reflection and Discussion

1. Discuss briefly the four components of nursing as a process and give a personal example to illustrate how this conceptual framework operates for you.

2. List five examples of technological advances that will be used in the future of health care delivery. How will these impact on the patient/client care that you will give?

3. What roles will the professional nurse play in the health prescriptive health system focus.

4. The future nurse manager must have a well internalized sense of self in order to promote excellent relationships with others. What can a nurse manager do to develop and foster this quality?

5. The policy-based function of professional nursing will change to standards defined. Review the American Nurses' Association generic standards of nursing practice and give reasons why they are so important to professional practice.

6. What is one of the most important factors assuring a well-prepared professional nurse in the future?

7. Describe the ideal hospital information system designed to support the business of health care in the marketplace. What role does the professional nurse have in this system?

8. What are the three essential ingredients in collaborative practice and why is this type of practice so critical to quality cost-effective care?

9. Do you believe nurses can develop entrepreneurial behaviors within your hospital and do you believe these behaviors would increase quality cost-effective patient care? Give reasons for your answers.

10. How critical is it that professional nurses play a central role in shaping health care delivery and what are the risks and benefits for these nurses?

REFERENCES

1. The Nature and Scope of Nursing Practice: Nursing: A Social Policy Statement. Kansas City, MO, American Nurses' Association, 1980
2. Bezold C: Health care in the U.S.: Four alternative futures. The Futurist 16:14–18, 1982
3. Naisbitt J: Megatrends. New York, Warner Books, 1982
4. Labor Letter: A Special News Report on People and Their Jobs in Offices, Fields, and Factories. Wall Streeet J May 27, 1986, p 1
5. Must hospitals form alliance to survive? Nurs Executive October 1986
6. Goldsmith J: 2036: A health care odyssey. Hospitals May 1986, pp 69–75.
7. Detmer SS: The future of health care delivery systems and settings. J Prof Nurs 2(1): 20–26, 1986
8. Lancaster J: 1986 and beyond, nursing's future. J Nurs Admin 16:25–37, 1986
9. Milio N: Telematics in the future of health care delivery: Implications for nursing. J Prof Nurs 2:39–50, 1986
10. Lutz L: Computers and health care. In Bezold C et al (eds): Pharmacy in the 21st Century. Alexandria, VA, Institute for Alternative Futures, 1985
11. Turner J: Computers, consumers, and pharmaceuticals. In Bezold C et al (eds): Pharmaceuticals in the Year 2000. Alexandria, VA, Institute for Alternative Futures, 1985
12. Dawson J: Can computers replace doctors? Private Practice June, 1983, pp 68–71.
13. Bezold C: The uncertain future: Alternative futures for the U.S. and health care. In Bezold C et al (eds): Pharmacy in the 21st Century. Alexandria, VA, Institute for Alternative Futures, 1985
14. Carlson R: Health care trends. In Bezold C et al (eds): Pharmacy in the 21st Century. Alexandria, VA, Institute for Alternative Futures, 1985
15. Porter–O'Grady T: Creative Nursing Administration: Participative Management into the 21st Century. Rockville, MD, Aspen Systems Corporation, 1986
16. Butler RN: A generation at risk. Across the Board July/August 1983, pp 37–45.

17. Roncoli M, Whitney F: The limits of medicine spell opportunities for nursing. Nurs Health Care 7(10):531–534, 1986
18. Curtin L: Nursing in the year 2000: Learning from the future. Nurs Man 17(6):7–8, 1986
19. Sovie M: Exceptional executive leadership shapes nursing's future. Nurs Economics 5(1):13–20, 1987
20. Hafer JC, Joiner C: Nurses as image emissaries: Are role conflicts impinging on a potential asset for an internal marketing strategy? J Health Care Marketing 4(1):25–35, 1984
21. Adelyotte MK: Nursing's preferred future. Nurs Outlook 35(3):119, 1987
22. Diers D: Preparation of practitioners, clinical specialists, and clinicians. J Prof Nurs 1(1):41–47, 1985
23. Mowry MM, Korpman RA: Evaluating automated information systems. Nurs Economics 5(1):7–12, 1987
24. Juran JM, Gryma FM Jr: Quality Planning and Analysis. New York, McGraw-Hill, 1970
25. Burchell RC, Thomas DA, Smith HL: Some considerations for implementing collaborative practice. Am J Med 74:9–13, 1983
26. Simms LM, Dalston JW, Roberts PW: Collaborative practice: Myth or reality? Hosp Health Services Admin 29:36–48, 1984
27. Ames A, Perrin JM: Collaborative practice: The joining of two professions. J Tenn Med Assoc 73(8):557–560, 1980
28. England DA: Collaboration in Nursing. Rockville, MD, Aspen Systems Corporation, 1986
29. Riley WJ, Schaefers V: Nursing operations as a profile center. Nurs Man 15(4):43–46, 1984

Index

ISBN 0-397-54649-1

90000